FRANCINE PRINCE'S
NEW DIET
FOR LIFE
COOKBOOK

FRANCINE PRINCE'S
NEW DIET
FOR LIFE
COOKBOOK

by

Francine Prince

A Perigee Book

For Harold

Perigee Books
are published by
The Putnam Publishing Group
200 Madison Avenue
New York, NY 10016

Copyright © 1990 by Francine Prince
All rights reserved. This book, or parts thereof,
may not be reproduced in any form without permission.
Published simultaneously in Canada

Library of Congress Cataloging-in-Publication Data

Prince, Francine.
    Francine Prince's new diet for life cookbook / by Francine Prince.
        p.   cm.
    Includes index.
    ISBN 0–399–51559–3
    1. Low-fat diet—Recipes.   2. Salt-free diet-Recipes.   3. Sugar-
free diet—Recipes.   I. Title.   II. Title: New diet for life
cookbook.
RM237.7.P75   1990
641.5′635—dc20   89–15960
                                                                      CIP

Printed in the United States of America
1 2 3 4 5 6 7 8 9 10

I would like to thank Lindley Boegehold, my editor, for her inestimable help in the preparation of this book, and Eugene Brissie, my publisher, for his continuing confidence in my work.

Contents

1
INTRODUCTION: THE *NEW* DIET FOR LIFE RECIPES

When my husband's cardiologist told him he would die if he walked a single block unless he agreed to triple-bypass surgery, he refused.

Harold said he would try an alternative way to recover from his heart attack.

Diet.

He told his doctor that the diet he intended to follow was very low in fat, saturated fat, and cholesterol, did not contain a grain of added salt or sugar, was stingy with calories, and high in fiber.

Harold, a Ph.D. in biochemistry, explained that according to some research findings, diet, plus exercise, could heal his clogged arteries and restore his health.

The doctor said he was crazy.

That was in 1974.

Today, more than fifteen years later, my husband is slim, vigorous, and in excellent health. He has never had surgery. And in all that time he has never taken a pill.

The secret of his recovery was the diet. But there was another secret, even more vital.

How he stayed on it.

He insisted at first on following cooking instructions conceived by nutrition scientists, and the food was a tasteless mess. Everything that makes food one of the joys of being alive—creaminess, sweetness, fattiness, saltiness, and the crunchy excitement of fried dishes—was achingly absent. The diet food tasted like cardboard or rubber. It sat in his stomach like cement. It was an ugly way to eat.

A few months after he went on the diet, he began to cheat.

But he wouldn't undergo surgery, and the diet was his only hope—a lifeline that was slowly unraveling.

"I had a problem," he jokes now. "And I handled it like a man. I handed it over to my wife."

But it was no joking matter then. What he expected me to do was to make healthy food taste good, and at that time nobody believed it could be done. Health-food advocates seemed to think that if food was medicine it should taste like medicine. In 1974, there were no guidelines for making healthy, tasty food.

I had to invent them. Time was running out, because Harold's cheating had escalated. Fortunately, I had the resources. I was brought up in the kitchen. I love to cook, to improvise, to create with my pots and pans. I was at that time a trained gourmet cook in the classic French style, and I had taken classes from a leading Chinese chef (with the aid of an interpreter). I had taught fine cooking, and I had learned from my students what Americans considered gourmet. I was ready.

It wasn't easy though. At first, there were failed dishes, disasters. But I never gave up. My husband's life was at stake, and the clock was running down. Then some dishes worked, then a few more, and overnight it seemed the food was good, very good. But even very good wasn't good enough. They had to be gourmet. I knew my husband, and he would settle for nothing less.

After a while, he didn't have to.

In about a year he was eating like a Prince.

That's another of his jokes.

But he never jokes when he says, "You saved my life."

I called my first collection of gourmet recipes for better health *The She Saved His Life Cookbook,* but my publisher thought the nation wasn't ready for that kind of claim (the year was 1979), and changed the title to *The Dieter's Gourmet Cookbook.* But the nation *was* ready for a haute cuisine of health, and the book was an instant success.

The following year I published *Diet for Life*—for the sake of your life. It contained a total nutritional program based on my husband's diet that included about a hundred new recipes—Diet for Life recipes. About a thousand more appeared in six subsequent books. All the recipes up to then were designed for people with special medical problems. One book, for example, was called *Francine Prince's Gourmet Recipes for Diabetics,* and its recipes were as austere in their nutritional demands as those for my husband's original diet.

Then something wonderful happened. In 1988, the U.S. Department of Health and Human Services issued its landmark "The Surgeon General's Report on Nutrition and Health." It gave my own work a totally new direction. No longer would my recipes be addressed to Americans on restricted diets, but to the great majority of Americans who were not. The new direction was mainstream—toward a healthier America.

And, thanks to the Report, my Diet for Life recipes would become even more attractive than before.

The Surgeon General's Report, according to Federal health officials, is the most comprehensive document on nutrition and health ever prepared by the government. The study took four years to prepare, involved the work of about 250 scientists, and is based on more than 2,500 research papers.

And yet the bottom line of the Report, in essence, is breathtakingly simple.

It tells most Americans that virtually nothing has to be cut completely from their diet.

It tells them instead to *cut down* on certain foods that are overconsumed, and *step up* on certain foods that are underconsumed.

And it tells them just what those foods are.

Foods to cut down on are those with excess fats, saturated fats, and cholesterol, as well as salt and sugar: hot dogs, French fries, ice cream, commercial hamburgers.

Foods to step up on have almost none of the above ingredients. These include fruits, vegetables, and grain products, plus lean meat, fish, chicken with skin removed, and fat-reduced dairy products. They're high in complex carbohydrates and dietary fiber.

Just cut down and step up—easy advice for anybody to follow.

It opened a new world of cooking opportunities for me. Remember, my Diet for Life recipes had a bare minimum of fat, saturated fat, and cholesterol, no salt, and zero sugar. I had nothing to cut down on. I could actually *add* some of those ingredients and get much the same, and frequently better, nutritional values than those people on an average American diet who were cutting down. I *could* add some fat, some salt, some cream, some sugar, some cholesterol foods—and what a scintillating difference even trifling amounts would make!

I had no concern about foods to step up on. I had used them from the time I had invented my first haute cuisine of health recipes. Now, they would be enriched with what Americans have long regarded as the can't-do-withouts of tastiness. The combination would be the basis of my *new* Diet for Life recipes—recipes for most Americans.

What are the cooking principles for the new Diet for Life recipes? There are just two:

· When you take tastes out, put tastes in.
· Use techniques, not just ingredients, to boost tastes.

I take tastes out when I cut down on foods from Dr. Koop's list of overconsumed foods. I put tastes in with the many ways that follow; and they are often more delicious than the tastes I take out.

The taste of fats. Cutting down on fats, Dr. Koop says, is the number-one dietary priority in the nation. But even at medically approved dietary levels, I'm able to evoke the flavor and succulence of fats with marinades and breadings in my meat, fish, and poultry dishes. Now that I can use small amounts of whole milk, light cream, and butter/ margarine blends to heighten flavor, some of my low-fat dishes taste like high-fat dishes.

But I don't use extra fat in most of my desserts and toppings. Evaporated (not condensed) skim milk is my base for an excellent ice cream and other glorious toppings.

The taste of cholesterol foods. Cholesterol, which chemically speaking, is not a fat and has no taste, is usually found in fatty animal foods. So, generally, when you cut down on fatty foods, you cut down on cholesterol—but it's the fatty *taste* that you miss. You can replace it as I've just described. But there's one cholesterol food whose taste you can't replace: the yolk of an egg.

Previously, I added an egg yolk (or a half yolk) as a flavoring in a recipe—if at all. Now I use a few more. If a recipe ordinarily calls for nine to twelve egg yolks (as it does for some baked goods), I use three. Even that relatively small amount becomes a sensational boon to taste.

Cholesterol watchers: Don't let those three egg yolks frighten you. In a cake that serves eight or more, the amount of cholesterol they contribute per serving is very, very little.

The taste of salt. Eliminating salt is a blessing in disguise. Instead of a single taste—salinity—I create a sparkling palette of flavors with mixes of herbs and spices, experiences that now peak when I add a pinch of salt to some of the mixes.

The taste of sugar. When sugar is absent, other ingredients—such as fruit, fruit juices and concentrates, cooked fruits, and sweet herbs and spices—endow my foods with a variety of confectionary flavors. Now, enriched with small amounts of sugar, foods have a sweetness that is new and wonderful.

How can techniques boost tastes? The following sampling of techniques (you'll find more as you go from recipe to recipe) demonstrates what a little vegetable oil can do in some cooking procedures to enhance taste and texture.

For searing in meat juices and flavors, I use a well-seasoned iron skillet. This is an invaluable utensil, superb for top-of-the-stove-to-oven cooking. It heats up to higher temperatures than the nonstick skillet, cooks foods faster, and turns out a much tastier meal. Cooking with an iron skillet requires some oil. (To prepare a well-seasoned iron skillet, see page 13.)

I use the nonstick skillet, which requires very little or no oil, for sautéing skinned chicken and thin-sliced meat and fish.

For tenderizing meats without using salty commercial tenderizers, you may want to use a clay pot, as I do in a couple of recipes. This ingenious cooking device turns out a tender, luscious dish. It requires just a little oil.

For giving foods that fried taste without frying, preheat the oven to high heat. Add small amounts of oil to a shallow metal baking pan (not aluminum; preferably stainless steel). Place in the oven for pre-scribed amount of time. Remove. Place breaded chicken in the pan. The quick searing of the meat creates the fried-chicken taste. (You can also use this technique with meats and fish.)

For a rich-tasting sauce for braised foods, transfer the meat, poultry, or fish to a serving plate after braising. Turn the heat up under the cooking utensil and reduce the sauce. It is now richly flavored, and has been thickened naturally by the vegetables in the sauce. If you prefer, you can then purée it in a blender or food processor to silken smoothness.

For a rich-tasting sauce for sautéed foods, reduce ingredients such as onions or shallots with vinegar and/or stock until only solids remain. *Then* add other liquids. This produces a vibrant sauce, utterly superior to the sauce produced from the same ingredients had they been only sautéed, then other liquids added.

And here's a technique that doesn't involve any oil at all: *For a saltier taste without adding more salt,* start the recipe with half the amount of salt called for. Add the rest at the last step.

The object of "The Surgeon General's Report on Nutrition and Health" is to bring healthful eating into the mainstream of American eating habits. It does this, Federal health officials assert, by providing the important scientific underpinnings for nutrition and health programs like my new Diet for Life cuisine. It transforms state-of-the-art nutrition into the art of fine cookery.

Fine cooking means dedication in the kitchen. This is not a quick-and-easy book. Nevertheless, preparation times and cooking times are reasonable, and most dishes can be ready within an hour. If you're already a cook, you know the joy of cooking—it's like no other joy in the world. If you're not a cook, you'll discover it when you begin making my Diet for Life meals.

Cooking is the best way to fulfill the promise of the Surgeon General's Report. There are no "magic muffins." The wide range of foods you need to help promote your family's good health is most easily, and most inexpensively, available from your grocery store and your oven. It's not necessary to cook every meal—that's impractical for most of us—but start with one dish, and you'll want to cook more. And more. I've prepared a Seven-Day Menu Plan (page 213) to help you make your selections.

For the statistic-watchers among you, I've charted the most recent government figures for recommended dietary allowances. My Menu

Plan matches some of them, betters others—particularly in salt control.

Most important, I've designed this book for food lovers. I've taken traditional delights and rephrased them in the contemporary culinary idiom. I've restored breadmaking to its joyous place in the kitchen. I've invented dishes that have no precedent to celebrate the birth of a healthy new American cuisine. For, thanks to the Surgeon General's keen, level-headed, authoritative advice on nutrition and health, this is a great time for celebration!

—Francine Prince

2

BEFORE YOU BEGIN

Here are a few hints on how to get the most from my new Diet for Life recipes.

· Read each recipe carefully before you start to cook. That includes the Notes and the Variations. The few extra minutes you spend on this will make your cooking go faster and more smoothly.

· All the herbs and spices I use are available in most supermarkets—except for saffron, which can be found in most gourmet grocery stores and finer supermarkets.

· Some of the recipes in this book require what I call My Basics (see Chapter 3). These are flavor aids that also speed up cooking. They'll perk up your own recipes too. Whenever they are called for in the list of ingredients, I have included the page in Chapter 3 where you'll find the specific recipe.

· All my breads freeze well. To keep loaves fresh-tasting for up to one month, follow this procedure: Wrap each loaf in plastic film, place in a paper bag, close, insert the paper bag into a plastic bag, seal tightly, and freeze. Defrost at room temperature for 1½ to 2 hours before slicing.

For instant toast, slice bread and then reassemble slices into a loaf. Freeze as described in the previous paragraph. When ready to use, just flick off slices and pop them into your toaster. There's no need to defrost.

Freeze breads and cakes prepared without yeast either whole or in serving pieces. Fifteen minutes before serving, rewrap in foil and bake in a preheated 400-degree oven, also for 15 minutes.

Recipes using a food processor have been tested with a large capacity unit (capable of managing up to 6 cups of flour).

· *To prepare a well-seasoned iron skillet,* wash the skillet in soapy water (do not soak it). Dry it thoroughly, then rub it sparingly with oil. Place the skillet over medium heat for three minutes. Let it cool. Wipe excess oil with paper toweling. Your skillet is now ready to use. After each use, simply wipe the skillet in soapy water with a sponge or cloth (do not use steel wool). Repeat this seasoning process whenever the skillet looks dry.

· For cornstarch thickening, be sure to prepare the mix just before using. To a full measure of cornstarch in a cup, stir in a small amount of liquid and repeat several times until the mix becomes completely smooth. Dribble just enough of mix into the sauce to thicken it to the consistency of light cream (or to your taste)—one to two tablespoons for a recipe serving four. It adds only about seven to fourteen calories per serving.

3
MY BASICS

SAVORY SEASONING

This piquant mixture of herbs and spices will transform any ordinary recipe into a very special dish. Unlike other flavor mixes, it never dominates, but swiftly blends in to heighten a recipe's essential taste. This handy seasoning is indispensable for soups, appetizers, main courses, and salads. To use, sprinkle it on foods *before* cooking, and add to salad dressings about 5 minutes before serving.

3 tablespoons onion powder
1 teaspoon each ground cinnamon and freshly grated nutmeg
1 tablespoon whole dried sage leaves, crushed, or 1 1/2 teaspoons rubbed sage
1/2 teaspoon dried thyme leaves, crushed

2 tablespoons each dried oregano, crushed, and mild curry powder
1 tablespoon ground ginger
5 whole cloves, crushed
1/4 teaspoon chili con carne seasoning
1/2 teaspoon salt (optional)

1. Combine all ingredients in a 1-cup jar. Stir to blend. Cover and shake several times.
2. Store, tightly closed, at room temperature. Stir gently with a spoon before each use.

Yield: **About 2/3 cup**

BOUQUET GARNI

A Bouquet Garni is a small bouquet of herbs whose delicate perfumes enrich the flavors of meats, poultry, soups, and stocks. It's an imperative of fine cooking.

For an average-size bundle you will need:
6 to 8 sprigs crisp fresh parsley, rinsed
1 small bay leaf ·
¼ teaspoon dried thyme leaves

For a large bundle you will need:
10 to 12 sprigs crisp fresh parsley, rinsed
1 large bay leaf
½ teaspoon dried thyme leaves

1. Lay parsley on a piece of paper toweling. Squeeze out water. Place parsley flat over a 5-inch-square piece of doubled washed *cotton* cheesecloth. Put bay leaf on top, and spoon thyme over it. (Use a larger piece of cheesecloth for the large Bouquet Garni, cutting away surplus to make a slim bundle.)
2. Fold up sides and tie securely with white cotton thread. Use whenever suggested in recipes throughout this book.

Yield: **1 bundle for each size Bouquet Garni.** Multiple bundles may be made and frozen *provided* cheesecloth is completely dry before filling. No defrosting is needed before using.

Note: Powdered thyme is not recommended for use in Bouquets Garnis.

BREADING MIX

When a recipe calls for "chicken with skin removed," here's a *second* skin to seal in the succulence. But the good news is that this skin is virtually free of fat and cholesterol! For a first-time effort, try making the mix for my Oven "Fried" Chicken (page 74) and see if you don't prefer the breading-mix chicken to a chicken fried in its own skin. You may also use Breading Mix as a coating for sautéed or baked fish or on well-trimmed meat.

3 tablespoons unhulled sesame seeds (available in health-food stores)
2 tablespoons oat bran
1 cup fine-toasted unseasoned bread crumbs, preferably homemade
1/4 cup each unbleached flour and stone-ground whole wheat flour
4 teaspoons stone-ground yellow

cornmeal
1 tablespoon onion powder
1/4 cup freshly grated Parmesan cheese (see Note*)*
1/2 teaspoon each mild curry powder, ground ginger, and ground cinnamon
1 teaspoon dried thyme leaves, crushed
1/4 teaspoon salt (optional)

1. Strew sesame seeds and oat bran across a small heated nonstick skillet. Over moderate heat, lightly toast seeds and bran, shaking skillet from time to time and taking care not to burn them. Let cool.
2. Combine remaining ingredients in medium-size bowl. Stir in seeds and bran.
3. Spoon mix into glass jar(s), but do not overfill (leave 2 inches from top). Stir or shake before using.

Yield: **About 2 1/4 cups. Recipe may be doubled.**

Variations:

1. When using on fish, add 1 teaspoon just-grated lemon zest for each 1/2 cup of mix.
2. For a spicy flavor, add 1/8 teaspoon cayenne pepper for each 1/2 cup of mix.

Note: Parmigiano Reggiano, a superior low-fat Parmesan cheese from Italy, will impart a superb flavor to this mix. It's generally available in fine cheese stores and gourmet food shops.

VEGETABLE MIX

When I want that extra zing to a dish, I often rely on this combination of garlic, shallots, and fresh ginger. I keep it on hand for instant cooking by freezing it flat in plastic-wrapped packets in 1-tablespoon measures. No defrosting is necessary. Just break it up and add to a hot skillet or saucepan.

*1 2-inch slice smooth-skinned fresh
    ginger (1-inch diameter)
5 large shallots, peeled and*
*   quartered
10 large cloves garlic, peeled and
    quartered*

1. Scrub ginger. If skin is not totally smooth, peel it away. Cut into ¼-inch slices.
2. Fit food processor with steel blade. With machine running, drop pieces through feed tube and process for 3 seconds. Then drop shallots and garlic through tube and process until mixture is fine-chopped to the size of pinheads. Store in freezer as described above.

Yield: **Scant cup**

Note: Following are the ingredients in smaller amounts and their approximate fine-chopped measurements. Use as a gauge when preparing smaller quantities of the mix. (An electric herb-chopper finely chops these ingredients in small amounts.)

Whole	Chopped
2 large cloves garlic	= 2 teaspoons
1 large shallot (1-inch diameter)	= 1 tablespoon
⅜-inch slice fresh ginger (1-inch diameter)	= 1½ teaspoons

CHICKEN STOCK

I can't conceive of cooking without Chicken Stock. Replete with the essence of chicken (and of meat bones, if a richer stock is desired), it can transmute the dullest recipe into a gastronomic feat. It's an intrinsic element in superb-tasting entrees, soups, and sauces.

1 3 1/2- to 4-pound broiling or
    stewing chicken (including
    neck and gizzard, but not the
    liver), skinned and quartered
2 pounds cracked veal and beef
    bones, well rinsed (optional)
4 ribs celery with leaves, cut into
    chunks
4 large cloves garlic, peeled and
    coarsely chopped
2 young carrots, peeled, cut into
    thick rounds
2 large leeks, split, well rinsed,
    ends trimmed, cut up
1 teaspoon grated fresh ginger
2 large snow-white fresh
    mushrooms, damp-wiped, ends
    trimmed, coarsely chopped
1 medium white turnip, trimmed,
    peeled, and cut into 1-inch
    cubes
4 whole cloves
1 large Bouquet Garni (page 16)
1/4 teaspoon dried dill weed
9 cups water

1. Place chicken, giblets, and bones in large heavy-bottomed kettle. Add celery, garlic, carrots, leeks, ginger, mushrooms, and turnip. Bring to boil. Cook for 2 minutes, skimming surface with large spoon as foam rises to top. Add remaining ingredients. Reduce heat to simmering. Cover (leave just a crack open) and cook for 2 1/2 hours, stirring from time to time.
2. Remove chicken and reserve for salads, sandwiches, or recipe for Cocktail Chicken Cabochons (pages 42–43). Pour ingredients through a sieve (a conical-shaped chinois is excellent for this task) into a bowl, pressing solids to extract juices. (If a strainer is used instead of a sieve, re-strain through a washed cotton cheese cloth.) Cover bowl and chill overnight.
3. Next day, cut away hardened fat that rises to the top (there won't be much). The stock is now ready to use. Store some in your refrigerator for use within 3 days, and freeze the balance in freeze-proof containers for up to 2 months.

Yield: **About 2 quarts**

Note: To keep small amounts handy, pour into ice-cube trays and freeze. Then transfer to double plastic bags. Each cube will contribute about 2 tablespoons of magic to your recipes.

VEGETABLE STOCK

This essence of fresh vegetables is a slightly sweet alternative to my Chicken Stock. The key word is *fresh,* for only vegetables that come to you as straight-from-the-farm as possible can yield the kind of bright, clean taste for which vegetable stock is noted. Use it whenever a recipe calls for my Vegetable Stock, or be adventurous and combine it with other stocks to create your own flavors.

2 medium carrots, peeled, cut into
    1-inch rounds
3/8-inch slice fresh ginger
3 ribs celery with leaves, trimmed,
    cut into 1-inch slices
2 medium onions, peeled, cut into
    1-inch chunks
1/2 medium butternut squash,
    peeled, seeded, pulp discarded,
    cut into 1-inch pieces
1 medium white turnip, trimmed,
    peeled, cut into 1-inch cubes

4 large cloves garlic, peeled and
    halved
1 1/2 cups canned unsalted Italian
    plum tomatoes
7 cups water
1 tablespoon white wine
    Worcestershire sauce
2 whole cloves
1/2 teaspoon each dried rubbed sage
    and mild curry powder
1/2 teaspoon salt
1 large Bouquet Garni (page 16)

1. Use food processor fitted with steel blade to fine-chop vegetables. Place carrots in workbowl. Cut ginger into 3 pieces. If skin is not smooth and unwrinkled, peel it off. Coarse-chop in on/off turns. Scrape into large heavy-bottomed kettle with cover.
2. Place celery and onions in workbowl; coarse-chop. Add to pot. Combine squash, turnip, and garlic in workbowl; coarse-chop. Scrape into pot.
3. Pour tomatoes into workbowl; process to a purée. Combine with vegetables in pot.
4. Add water and Worcestershire sauce to pot. Bring to boil, skimming surface with large spoon as foam rises to top.
5. Add all remaining ingredients except salt. Bring to boil; reduce heat to simmering. Cover (leave a crack open) and simmer for 1 1/2 hours, stirring from time to time.
6. With bowl underneath, pour stock through a fine sieve or a strainer lined with a piece of washed cotton cheesecloth. Sprinkle in salt, stirring until dissolved.
7. When completely cooled, refrigerate stock in tightly closed 1-quart jar for up to 4 days. Stir before using. Place balance in freeze-proof

containers for up to 2 months. For another storage hint, see the *Note* for Chicken Stock (page 19).

Yield: **About 7 cups**

FISH STOCK

This stock, crucial to sauces accompanying well-prepared fish dishes, is the easiest of all stocks to prepare (only a few simple steps), the quickest (just 30 minutes cooking time), and the most economical (your fishmonger will be glad to *give* you the bones). But the seasoning it imparts seems to come from a four-star chef who frets over his work. For exceptional results, use red snapper or Dover sole carcasses when available.

3 pounds fish bones and heads (from white flat fish), cut up
1 tablespoon Italian olive oil
2 tablespoons Vegetable Mix (page 18) or equivalent ingredients
2 ribs celery with leaves, sliced
1 onion, coarsely chopped
2 large snow-white fresh mushrooms, ends trimmed,
damp-wiped, and coarsely chopped
1/2 cup dry white wine
5 1/2 cups water
1-inch slice lemon peel
2 whole cloves
10 peppercorns
1 Bouquet Garni (page 16)

1. Rinse fish bones and heads under cold running water. Drain and reserve.
2. Heat oil in large heavy-bottomed saucepan or kettle until hot. Add Vegetable Mix, celery, and onion. Sauté over moderate heat until softened (about 6 minutes). Stir in mushrooms and sauté for 1 minute longer.
3. Add bones. Raise heat. Turn bones over in pan until coated with sauteed ingredients, cooking them for 3 minutes.
4. Add wine. Bring to boil. Then add water and remaining ingredients. Bring to boil again, skimming the surface occasionally as foam rises to top. Reduce heat to simmering. Cook, uncovered, for about 30 minutes until liquid is reduced to 4½ cups.
5. Pour stock through a sieve, pressing out juices. Refrigerate in well-covered bowl for 1 day. Skim off thin layer of fat. Store in 1-cup containers for up to 1 month.

Yield: **About 4½ cups. Recipe doubles successfully.**

CANNED STOCK PERK-UP

When your supply of my Chicken Stock runs low, haul unsalted canned chicken stock or beef broth from your larder and perk up their blandness with this simple recipe. The wonderful surprise is: It works very well—that is, until you have a chance to make more of the real thing.

2 13¾-ounce cans unsalted
    chicken or beef broth
½ teaspoon instant (freeze-dried)
    minced garlic
3 cloves, crushed
½ teaspoon each mild curry

    powder and dried dill weed
2 teaspoons onion powder
2 medium snow-white fresh
    mushrooms, damp-wiped,
    trimmed, and sliced
1 Bouquet Garni (page 16)

1. Combine all ingredients in heavy-bottomed saucepan. Bring to boil. Reduce heat to simmering. Cover partially and simmer for 15 minutes. Let cool.
2. Strain stock through a sieve. Store in refrigerator in a tightly covered jar for up to 3 days. Stir before using.

Yield: **About 3 cups**

Variation: Substitute 1 tablespoon Savory Seasoning (page 15) for cloves, curry, dill, and onion powder.

TOMATO SAUCE

I freeze this robust tomato sauce in 1-cup measures in boilable bags for an almost-instant pasta dinner, and whenever I want real tomato flavor in any recipe.

2 small tender ribs celery, strings
    pulled off
1 each medium sweet red and green
    pepper
1 large onion, peeled
4 large cloves garlic, peeled and
    halved
1 28-ounce can unsalted Italian
    plum tomatoes

2 tablespoons Italian olive oil
2 teaspoons dried oregano, crushed
1 teaspoon each ground ginger and
    curry powder
1/8 teaspoon salt
1 tablespoon red wine vinegar
1 tablespoon unsalted tomato paste
1/2 teaspoon sugar
1 Bouquet Garni (page 16)

1. Fit food processor with steel blade. Cut celery, peppers, and onion into 1-inch pieces; halve each garlic clove. Place all in workbowl of food processor and coarsely chop, turning on/off 4 to 5 times. Transfer to bowl, add tomatoes, and purée until smooth.

2. Heat oil in a 2-quart heavy-bottomed saucepan until hot. Add chopped mixture. Sprinkle with seasonings and sauté until softened, about 5 minutes, stirring often.

3. Add vinegar. Cook for 1 minute. Then add puréed tomatoes, tomato paste, sugar, and bouquet garni. Bring to a boil. Reduce heat to a simmer. Cover and cook at a steady simmer for 1 hour, stirring from time to time and adjusting heat when necessary. Discard bouquet garni after pressing out juices. Use immediately, or let cool before packaging for freezer.

Yield: **4½ to 5 cups. Recipe doubles successfully.**

4

SOUPS AND STARTERS

ORANGE BROCCOLI SOUP

This is a subtle vegetable soup. Although broccoli is the main ingredient, the stock and orange juice keep it from dominating the flavor of the soup. Imported short-grain rice is the natural thickener.

4 cloves garlic, peeled
1 large onion, peeled
4 cups fresh broccoli florets,
    including 1 inch of stem
    (about 1 small bunch)
1/4 pound snow-white fresh
    mushrooms, ends trimmed,
    damp-wiped
1 tablespoon Italian olive oil
1/4 cup Arborio rice, rinsed (see
    Note)

1 1/2 teaspoons dried tarragon
    leaves, crumbled
1 teaspoon mild curry powder
2 1/2 cups Chicken or Vegetable
    Stock (pages 19–21)
1 cup fresh orange juice
1/2 cup evaporated skim milk
3 tablespoons light cream
Freshly ground black pepper
1/4 teaspoon salt
Freshly grated Parmesan cheese

1. Fit food processor with steel blade. Cut garlic into quarters and onion into 1-inch chunks. Add to workbowl. Fine-chop with 5 or 6 on/off turns; scrape into a measuring cup. (You will need 1 cup.) Coarse-chop broccoli with 4 to 5 on/off turns. Transfer to plate. Quarter each mushroom and fine-chop in 4 to 5 on/off turns.
2. Heat oil in heavy-bottomed 3-quart saucepan. Sauté garlic and onion over medium heat for 2 minutes, taking care not to brown. Scrape mushrooms into saucepan and sauté for 2 minutes. Add rice, stirring several times to coat. Then add broccoli, sprinkle in seasonings, and sauté for 1 minute.
3. Add stock and orange juice. Bring to boil. Reduce heat to simmering, cover, and simmer for 30 minutes, stirring every 10 minutes.
4. Remove from heat. Add milk, cream, pepper, and salt. Reheat to just under simmering, then ladle into serving bowls. Serve Parmesan on the side.

Yield: **Serves 6**

GOLDEN CARROT SOUP WITH SHRIMP

This is *not* a typical sweet carrot soup. The addition of turnip, spices, and shrimp gives it a new, sophisticated taste. Choose medium or small shrimp—they're sweeter, and are less likely than larger ones to become chewy when cooked in liquid. Also, you'll get more shrimp per pound because the shells are thinner.

1 pound fresh long slender carrots, trimmed, peeled, cut into ½-inch cubes
1 medium white turnip, trimmed, peeled, cut into ½-inch cubes
3 cups Chicken Stock (page 19)
2 medium leeks, white part only
1 tablespoon Vegetable Mix (page 18), or equivalent amounts of fresh ginger, garlic, and shallot
2 teaspoons Italian olive oil
½ teaspoon each freshly grated nutmeg, ground cardamom, and ginger

2 tablespoons fresh lemon juice
1 Bouquet Garni—made with 4 sprigs of dill instead of parsley (page 16)
1 cup low-fat milk (1% milk fat)
3 tablespoons light cream
½ pound small fresh shrimp, shelled, deveined, each cut into thirds
¼ teaspoon salt
2 teaspoons sugar (optional)
1 tablespoon minced just-snipped fresh dill
Freshly ground white or black pepper

1. Place carrots and turnip in steamer. Cover and steam until firm-tender (do not overcook). Transfer to workbowl of food processor that has been fitted with steel blade. Add ¼ cup Chicken Stock. Purée until very smooth (about 1½ minutes), stopping machine and scraping down sides of workbowl when necessary. Turn into another bowl. Rinse out workbowl.
2. Trim leeks, discarding thick outer skin; slit down center rinse under cold running water. Cut into 1-inch slices. Drop into workbowl and fine-mince. There should be ½ cup. If you're not using prepared Vegetable Mix, mince the equivalents now.
3. Heat oil in heavy-bottomed 3-quart saucepan. Over moderate heat, sauté leeks and Vegetable Mix until tender; do not brown. Sprinkle with spices. Stir and cook for 1 minute. Pour in remaining 2¾ cups stock, puréed vegetables, and lemon juice. Drop in the bouquet garni. Bring to a boil. Reduce heat, partially cover, and simmer for 30 minutes. Add milk and cream and continue to simmer for 5 more minutes.

4. Raise heat. Add shrimp and salt. When soup comes back to a simmer, reduce heat slightly and cook, uncovered, for 3 minutes. Taste. Add sugar, if desired. Discard bouquet garni after pressing out juices. Serve sprinkled with dill and freshly ground pepper in warm bowls.

Yield: **Serves 5**

PUMPKIN SOUP

The cooking time is brief (plain canned pumpkin is your kitchen-quick ally) for this thick puree, enriched with a mélange of vegetables and zesty spices.

2 large onions
2 large shallots
1 large rib celery
1 large carrot
1 tablespoon each walnut oil and sweet butter/margarine blend
2 teaspoons mild curry powder
1/2 teaspoon each cinnamon and dried mint leaves
1 1/2 cups unsweetened apple juice

1 cup Chicken Stock (page 19)
1 16-ounce can solid-pack pumpkin
1 large Bouquet Garni (page 16), including 4 whole cloves
1 cup milk
1/2 cup evaporated skim milk
1/4 teaspoon salt (optional)
Freshly ground black pepper
Minced parsley

1. Fit food processor with steel blade. Cut onions, shallots, celery, and carrot into 1-inch pieces, place in workbowl, and process with about 5 on/off turns to coarse-chop.
2. Heat oil and shortening in heavy-bottomed 3-quart saucepan until hot. Over medium-high heat, sauté chopped mixture for 1 minute. Sprinkle with spices and mint and continue sautéeing until vegetables are limp but not brown (about 4 minutes).
3. Stir in apple juice and stock. Bring to boil. Then whisk in pumpkin. Add bouquet garni, reduce heat to simmering, cover, and simmer for 25 minutes. Let stand, partially covered, in pot for 10 minutes. Discard Bouquet Garni after pressing out juices.
4. Puree in two batches in food processor or blender until very smooth. Pour back into saucepan. Whisk in milks, salt, and pepper. Reheat to just under boiling point. Serve at once with garnish of parsley.

Yield: **Serves 6 to 7**

SUMMER AND WINTER SQUASH SOUP

I've combined zucchini (a summer squash) with butternut squash (a winter variety) and produced a new satiny-smooth soup. Both vegetables are available most of the year. Prepare them in this soup to add a sparkling fresh taste to your luncheon or dinner menu.

1 tablespoon Italian olive oil
2 medium onions, cut into 1/2-inch chunks
2 medium shallots, quartered
1 cup 1-inch cubed butternut squash
2 cups well-scrubbed zucchini, cut in 1-inch cubes
1 crisp apple (such as Washington State), peeled, cored, and coarsely chopped
1/4 cup Arborio rice, rinsed (see Note)

1 teaspoon each mild curry powder and ground cinnamon
1/2 teaspoon anise seed
2 cups Vegetable Stock (page 20)
6 sprigs parsley, rinsed, wrapped into neat bundle with white cotton thread
1 cup low-fat buttermilk, preferably without salt
1/4 teaspoon salt
1 tablespoon minced parsley or fresh mint
Freshly ground white pepper

1. Heat oil in heavy-bottomed 3-quart saucepan. Add onions and shallots. Sauté over moderate heat until wilted (about 5 minutes), stirring often.
2. Stir in butternut squash, zucchini, apple, and rice. Sauté for 2 minutes, stirring to coat. Sprinkle in spices and anise seed. Add stock and parsley bundle. Bring to a boil. Reduce heat to simmering. Cook for 30 minutes, stirring twice at equal intervals. Uncover partially and let soup cool for 5 minutes. Discard parsley bundle after pressing out juices.
3. Purée in food blender in two batches. Pour soup back into rinsed-out saucepan. Stir in buttermilk, salt, and parsley or mint. Heat to just below simmering point. Serve at once, sprinkled with pepper, in warmed soup bowls.

Yield: **Serves 5 to 6**

Note: Arborio is a short-grained Italian rice that is a fine natural thickener. It's available in fine gourmet shops and Italian grocery stores.

POTATO SOUP WITH FENNEL

Fennel's strong licorice flavor is tamed to delicacy when it is cooked longer than 2 minutes, especially with flavor-absorbing potatoes, as it is here. That combination is then fused with stock, sweet and tart fruits, and buttermilk to create a wintertime soup that's heart- and body-warming.

*1 small fennel bulb, including 2
   inches of stem and some of
   the feathery fronds, cut into
   1-inch pieces*
*¼ cup loosely packed parsley
   florets*
*1 medium onion, cut into 1-inch
   pieces*
3 large cloves garlic, quartered
*1½ pounds Idaho potatoes, peeled,
   cut into 2-inch chunks*
*1 medium Golden Delicious apple,
   peeled, cored, and quartered*

*1½ tablespoons peanut oil or
   Italian olive oil*
1½ teaspoons mild curry powder
*¼ teaspoon each cinnamon and
   freshly grated nutmeg*
*2 cups Chicken or Vegetable Stock
   (pages 19, 20)*
¼ cup unsweetened apple juice
Pinch cayenne pepper
¼ teaspoon salt
2 tablespoons fresh lemon juice
*¾ cup low-fat buttermilk,
   preferably unsalted*

1. Fit food processor with steel blade. Put fennel, parsley, onion, and garlic in workbowl. Process until fine-chopped (about 10 seconds). Scrape into measuring cup. You will need 2 cups; if you have less, add more fine-chopped onion. Process potatoes in 4 on/off turns until they are about ½-inch pieces. Transfer to plate. Cut each apple-quarter into thirds and fine-chop in 6 on/off turns. Add to potatoes.
2. Heat oil in heavy-bottomed 3-quart saucepan. Sauté fennel mixture over moderate heat until softened without browning (about 4 minutes). Stir in potatoes and apples. Sprinkle with spices and cook for 2 minutes, stirring continually.
3. Add stock, apple juice, and a sprinkling of cayenne pepper. Bring to boil. Reduce heat to simmering. Cover and simmer for 25 minutes, stirring often. Mixture will be thick.
4. Sprinkle in salt and lemon juice and combine. Gradually stir in buttermilk. Heat until just under simmering, maintaining constant heat for 5 minutes. Ladle into warmed soup bowls and serve at once.

Yield: **Serves 6**

Note: If Vegetable Stock is used, eliminate apple juice and increase stock to 2¼ cups.

GREEN PEA AND WATERCRESS SOUP

Ever since I first visited Paris, I've been in love with petit pois—so tiny, sweet, and tender. In those halcyon days, I ordered them, or a soup made from them, with every meal except breakfast. My version of a green pea soup is frugal with salt, but extravagant with spices, herbs, bitter-edged with watercress, and enriched with stock. If you can't find tiny fresh peas, good-quality frozen ones make a beautiful soup too.

1 tablespoon Italian olive oil
1/2 cup coarsely chopped scallions, including 2 inches green part below bulb, trimmed, tough outer skin discarded
2 tablespoons coarsely chopped shallots
1 tightly packed cup crisp watercress leaves (about one large bunch), rinsed
2 1/2 cups Chicken or Vegetable Stock (pages 19, 20), or a

combination of both
1 teaspoon dried tarragon leaves
1 teaspoon mild curry powder
1/4 teaspoon salt
2 cups shelled tiny fresh green peas, or one 10-ounce box frozen tiny green peas
1/2 cup milk
2 tablespoons cream (optional)
1/4 teaspoon freshly grated nutmeg
Pinch cayenne pepper

1. Pour oil into medium heavy-bottomed saucepan. Over moderate heat, sauté scallions and shallots until limp. Stir in watercress; sauté for 1 minute. Add 1 cup stock, tarragon, curry powder, salt, and peas. Bring to boil. Reduce heat to simmering. Cover and cook gently until peas are tender (frozen peas will cook more rapidly than fresh).
2. With slotted spoon, transfer solids to workbowl of food processor fitted with steel blade. Add 1/4 cup soup liquid to workbowl. Process until well puréed. Then add remaining soup liquid to workbowl and process until well blended.
3. Pour back into rinsed-out saucepan. Stir in remaining 1 1/2 cups stock, milk, cream, and nutmeg. Bring to simmering point. Gently cook, uncovered, for 5 minutes. Ladle into warmed individual soup bowls and serve at once.

Yield: **Serves 4 to 5**

YAM BISQUE

Yams, which are *not* sweet potatoes, are a winter-holiday food (usually), served with marshmallows (usually). I'm on a one-woman campaign to rectify that indignity. Yams deserve gourmet treatment, and they deserve it all year round.

4 large shallots, quartered
1 medium yam, peeled
2 medium carrots, peeled and
     trimmed
2 medium cucumbers, peeled and
     trimmed
2 ribs celery, trimmed
Florets from 10 sprigs Italian flat
     parsley
2 tablespoons Italian olive oil
1 tablespoon curry powder
1 tablespoon dried rosemary,

     crushed
1 tablespoon balsamic vinegar
2 cups Chicken Stock (page 19) or
     Vegetable Stock (page 20)
1/8 teaspoon salt
1 tablespoon regular cream of
     wheat
1/4 cup plain low-fat yogurt, or 2
     tablespoons each yogurt and
     Light Choice sour cream (see
     Note)
2 tablespoons minced chives

1. Fit food processor with steel blade. Place shallots in workbowl and fine-mince. Scrape into cup. Cut yam and carrots into 1-inch chunks. Drop into workbowl and coarsely chop. Scrape into bowl.
2. Cut cucumbers and celery into 1-inch slices. Place in workbowl with parsley florets. Process on/off 4 times.
3. Heat oil in heavy-bottomed 3-quart saucepan. Add shallots and sauté over medium heat for 1 minute. Stir in curry powder and cook for 1 minute. Combine balance of chopped ingredients and rosemary; cook for 2 minutes.
4. Pour in vinegar. Cook for 30 seconds, stirring to combine. Add stock and salt. Cook, covered, over medium heat for 30 minutes.
5. Purée through food mill and pour back into saucepan. Bring to simmering point. While stirring, sprinkle with cream of wheat and cook for 10 minutes. Soup will thicken slightly. Stir in yogurt or sour cream. Ladle into soup dishes and top with chives.

Yield: **Serves 5**

Note: Light Choice is a low-fat sour cream manufactured by Breakstone's and tastes very much like the real thing.

HEARTY VEGETABLE SOUP WITH CHICKEN

Replete with dried mushrooms, barley, tender chicken morsels, and concentrated tomato sauce, this stock-enriched soup makes a hearty entree. It's high in fiber, too.

1/2 ounce imported dried mushrooms, dark variety (see Note)

1 cup boiling water

3/4 pound boned and skinned chicken breasts, cut into bite-size pieces

1 teaspoon each mild curry and rubbed sage leaves

1 1/2 tablespoons Italian olive oil

1 1/2 tablespoons minced garlic

1/4 cup barley

1 tablespoon unbleached flour

1 1/2 cups Chicken Stock (page 19)

2 1/2 cups Tomato Sauce (page 23)

3 tablespoons coarsely chopped parsley

1/4 teaspoon salt

3 to 4 tablespoons freshly grated Parmesan cheese

1. Rinse mushrooms; break them up and place in small bowl. Stir in boiling water. Let stand for 30 minutes. Pour mixture through strainer, pressing out juices into bowl. Fine-chop mushrooms; reserve soaking liquid.

2. Place chicken pieces in bowl. Sprinkle with seasonings and combine well.

3. Heat oil in heavy-bottomed 3-quart saucepan. Over moderate heat, sauté garlic for 1 minute. Add chopped mushrooms; sauté for 30 seconds. Raise heat slightly and sauté chicken with mixture until it loses its raw look (about 4 minutes). Strew barley into saucepan and cook for 1 minute.

4. Sprinkle with flour. Stir and cook for 1 minute. Then add reserved mushroom liquid, stock, tomato sauce, and parsley and bring to a boil. Reduce heat to simmering, cover and cook for 50 minutes, stirring 3 times at equal intervals. Stir in salt. Re-cover and let stand for 10 minutes before serving. Heat soup over moderate heat for 1 minute.

5. Ladle into warmed bowls. Sprinkle with Parmesan and serve very hot.

Yield: **Serves 5**

Note: These mushrooms are labeled "Imported Dried Mushrooms" and are available in supermarkets. They are packed in 1/2-ounce clear plastic boxes for easy identification of the light or dark variety.

LENTIL AND BEAN SOUP

Fiber means more than bran and more bran. Beans and legumes are high in fiber and can also help lower cholesterol. Don't pass this one by if you're one of the multitude who has always complained "I can't eat beans!"

1/3 cup each pinto beans and
   brown lentils
1/2 ounce imported dry mushrooms,
   preferably the dark variety
1 medium onion, peeled
4 large shallots, peeled
2 ribs celery, trimmed
1 small sweet green pepper, seeded
1 small white turnip, peeled and
   trimmed

3 large cloves garlic, peeled
4 teaspoons Savory Seasoning
   (page 15)
2 tablespoons balsamic vinegar
3 1/2 cups Chicken Stock (page 19)
1/4 cup coarsely chopped flat
   Italian parsley leaves
pinch cayenne pepper
1/8 to 1/4 teaspoon salt

1. Put beans and lentils in strainer. Pick over; rinse under cold running water for 1 minute and drain. Place in bowl, cover with cold water and soak for 1 hour, then drain. Add fresh water and repeat procedure once more. Soak for 2 hours (or overnight if you have difficulty digesting beans).

2. Rinse mushrooms. Break up, place in cup, barely cover with boiling water, and let soak.

3. Chop vegetables by hand or use food processor. To use processor, cut onion into 1-inch chunks. Halve shallots. Fit food processor with steel blade and process on/off until coarsely chopped. Scrape onto plate and set aside. Cut celery, green pepper, and turnip into 1-inch chunks; halve garlic cloves. Process on/off until coarsely chopped.

4. Heat oil in heavy-bottomed 3-quart saucepan until very hot. Sauté onion and shallots over medium-high heat, stirring continually until lightly browned. Add celery mix and combine. Sprinkle with Savory Seasoning and sauté over moderate heat for 5 minutes.

5. Mix vinegar into ingredients. Cook for 2 minutes. Stir in stock and parsley. Pour soaked beans into strainer. Rinse under cold running water for 30 seconds. Add to saucepan and bring to boil. Reduce heat to simmering, cover, and cook for 1 1/2 hours, stirring from time to time.

6. Stir in cayenne pepper and salt. Re-cover and cook for 5 minutes. Remove from heat and let stand for 5 minutes before serving.

Yield: **Serves 5**

Serving suggestion: Green salad and thin-sliced Masterpiece Bread (page 156) are perfect accompaniments.

THICK CABBAGE SOUP WITH WILD RICE

As a small child, I never liked soup. Except cabbage soup. It was prepared in our home from a very fatty cut of meat, with coarse chunks of cabbage and scads of sugar counterpointed with lemon juice. Delicious, but unhealthy. My version uses a lean cut of meat, hand-sliced cabbage, a bit of sugar, lemon juice, sweet tarragon, and various seasonings. Plus wild rice!

1 1/2 pounds beef hind shank, bone-in, well trimmed of fat and gristle
3/4 teaspoon each cinnamon and ground ginger
1 1/2 teaspoons crumbled dry tarragon
1/2 teaspoon salt
2 tablespoons Italian olive oil
1 cup coarsely chopped onion
2 teaspoons minced garlic
1 medium cabbage (1 3/4 pounds), cored, coarse outer leaves discarded, coarsely chopped

1/4 cup wild rice, rinsed
1 large, crisp sweet apple, such as Washington State, cored, peeled, and coarsely chopped
1 tablespoon balsamic vinegar
3 cups unsalted canned beef broth, or 1 1/2 cups each Chicken Stock (page 19) and water
3 cups unsalted Italian plum tomatoes, coarsely chopped
1/2 cup fresh lemon juice
1 tablespoon sugar
1 Bouquet Garni (page 16)

1. Cut meat from bone. Slice into bite-size pieces. In cup, combine spices, tarragon, and salt. Sprinkle and rub half of mixture over meat.
2. Heat oil in heavy-bottomed 3-quart kettle until hot. Sauté onion and garlic over moderate heat until wilted but not brown. Add meat and cook until it loses its pink color. Combine cabbage with mixture (volume will decrease as it steams). Add bone. Cook for 5 minutes, stirring with a large spoon every minute. Add rice and apple. Continue cooking and stirring for 2 minutes.
3. Pour vinegar around sides of pot. Combine and cook for 2 minutes. Add beef broth (or alternative), tomatoes, lemon juice, and sugar. Drop in Bouquet Garni. Bring to a boil, then reduce heat to simmering. Cover and simmer for 2 1/2 hours, stirring from time to time.
4. Remove from heat and let stand for 5 minutes. Discard bone and Bouquet Garni. Pour soup into warmed tureen, and serve.

Yield: **Serves 8**

Variation: Stir in 2 tablespoons Light Choice sour cream or plain low-fat yogurt just before serving.

CELERY ROOT SOUP

Despite its name, celery root is *not* celery. Sometimes called celerial or knob celery, it's a root vegetable with a fibrous peel. Its flavor is especially aromatic. Particularly so when paired with potato and sparked with pungent dried rosemary and curry, as it is here.

2 teaspoons fresh lemon juice
Water
1 1/2 pounds untrimmed celery root, deep-peeled, cut into 1/2-inch cubes
1 tablespoon Italian olive oil
2 tablespoons Vegetable Mix (page 18)
1/2 cup coarsely chopped onion
1 teaspoon each dried rosemary leaves, crushed, and mild

curry powder
2 cups Chicken Stock (page 19)
1 1/4 cups Tomato Sauce (page 23)
1 medium Idaho potato, cut into 1/2-inch cubes (1 cup)
1/4 cup tightly packed parsley florets
1/8 to 1/4 teaspoon salt
2 to 3 tablespoons Light Choice sour cream
Minced parsley

1. Place lemon juice in medium bowl. Fill three-quarters with water. Drop celery root into liquid as it's cut to prevent discoloration.
2. Heat oil in heavy-bottomed 3-quart saucepan. Sauté Vegetable Mix and onion until softened without browning. Stir in rosemary and curry powder. Cook over moderate heat for 30 seconds. Add stock, Tomato Sauce, potato, and parsley florets. Drain celery root and add to pot. Bring to boil, reduce heat to simmering, then cover and gently simmer for 30 minutes. Partially uncover and let cool for 10 minutes.
3. Purée in batches in food blender. Mixture will be thick. Re-warm over low heat. Whisk in salt and 2 tablespoons sour cream, adding remaining tablespoon if desired. Serve, sprinkled with parsley, in warmed bowls. (Reheat chilled leftovers in double boiler.)

Yield: **Serves 6**

Variations:

1. One cup Italian tomato purée (unsalted) may be substituted for 1 1/4 cups of Tomato Sauce. The flavor won't be quite the same, but it works.
2. Plain low-fat yogurt may be substituted for the sour cream. Add 1/2 teaspoon sugar when reheating.

SUN-DRIED TOMATO TART

This is a delicious, Provence-inspired food. The filling is a mix of sun-dried tomatoes, mushrooms, reduced onions, garlic, and stock. The cookie-textured shell features rolled oats. The ensemble is wholesome and scrumptious—a far cry from yesterday's egg- and cream-based quiche.

For the filling:

1 cup firmly packed sun-dried tomatoes, rinsed
Boiling water
1 1/2 tablespoons Italian olive oil
2 cups coarsely chopped onions
2 tablespoons coarsely chopped garlic
1 tablespoon red wine vinegar
1 cup Chicken Stock (page 19) or canned unsalted beef broth
2 tablespoons coarsely chopped flat parsley
1/2 teaspoon dried tarragon leaves, crumbled

1/4 teaspoon freshly grated nutmeg
1/4 pound snow-white fresh mushrooms
2 teaspoons prepared Dijon mustard, preferably without salt
2 tablespoons Light Choice sour cream or plain low-fat yogurt
3/4 cup grated part-skim mozzarella (do not pack)
1 1/2 teaspoons melted sweet butter/margarine blend
3 tablespoons chopped chives

For the crust:

1/4 cup rolled oats
1 cup unbleached flour, spooned into measuring cup and leveled off with knife
1/4 teaspoon salt
1/2 teaspoon non-aluminum baking powder

1/4 teaspoon each ground coriander and freshly grated nutmeg
3 tablespoons light cream cheese (Neufchâtel)
2 tablespoons Italian olive oil
3 to 4 tablespoons hot tap water

1. Prepare filling first. Place tomatoes in small bowl. Pour enough boiling water over them to barely cover. Let soften for 20 minutes. Drain. Partially squeeze out and chop coarsely. Set aside.

2. Heat oil in medium heavy-bottomed saucepan. Add onions and garlic. Sauté over medium heat until lightly browned, stirring often (about 7 minutes). Stir in vinegar; cook for 1 minute. Add stock and parsley. Bring to a boil. Reduce heat to simmering and cook, uncovered, until liquid is reduced by half.

3. Sprinkle in tarragon and nutmeg. Damp-wipe mushrooms; trim ends. Cut each mushroom in half and then thin-slice crosswise. Add to mixture, blending well. Simmer, uncovered, until liquid evaporates, taking care not to scorch. Cooking is completed when medley is moist without any running liquid. Stir in tomatoes, mustard, and sour cream.

4. To prepare pastry, fit food processor with steel blade. Place oats in workbowl and pulverize. Add flour, salt, baking powder, and spices. Process for 10 seconds. Uncover workbowl, drop pieces of cream cheese into workbowl, re-cover, and process for 4 seconds. Then pour oil through feed tube and process for 6 seconds. With machine running, dribble water through feed tube, 1 tablespoon at a time, until dough forms soft spongy balls (4 tablespoons usually does it).

5. Preheat oven to 350 degrees.

6. Moisten work surface. Cover with sheet of wax paper. Scoop up dough and shape into ball. Place on paper. With heel of hand, press into a smooth 8-inch circle. Cover with another sheet of paper. Gently roll dough between both sheets to a 12-inch circle. Gingerly remove top sheet of paper. Lift up bottom sheet with dough, invert, and ease into an 8-inch pie pan. Trim any ragged edges. Fold under edge and press to lip of pan, leaving a generous band. Chill for 15 minutes.

7. Spoon half the filling into shell. Sprinkle with half the mozzarella. Spoon remaining filling over mozzarella, smoothing it out. Sprinkle with remaining mozzarella.

8. Bake in center section of oven for 20 minutes. Brush crust and filling with melted shortening and return to oven for 5 minutes. Place on rack. Immediately sprinkle with chives. Serve warm.

Yield: **Serves 8**

PINTO BEAN CAKES

These little bean cakes resemble croquettes but they're *uncoated* and *sautéed* in a smidgen of fat. They're a modern, healthy hors d'oeuvre.

3/4 cup dried pinto beans
1/4 teaspoon salt
1/2 small carrot, peeled, cut into
    1/4-inch rounds
2 large shallots, quartered
1/4 cup each loosely packed
    coriander leaves and parsley
    florets, rinsed
1/2 teaspoon each cumin and
    ground ginger
2 tablespoons Chicken Stock (page
    19) or Vegetable Stock (page
    20)
1/2 teaspoon Worcestershire sauce
2 teaspoons Italian olive oil

2 tablespoons unbleached flour
1/4 teaspoon non-aluminum baking
    powder
2 tablespoons minced boiled ham
1/4 teaspoon freshly ground black
    pepper
About 1 1/2 tablespoons Italian
    olive oil
1 bunch arugula, well rinsed and
    dried
Fresh lemon juice
Lemon wedges
1 Kirby cucumber, peeled and
    thin-sliced

1. Pour beans into strainer; pick over and rinse under cold running water. (See instructions for soaking in Step 1 of Lentil and Bean Soup, page 33.) Drain last soaking liquid. Place beans in heavy-bottomed 1¾-quart saucepan. Fill pan three-quarters full with water and bring to a boil. Sprinkle in salt. Reduce heat to simmering. Cover and simmer until tender (45 to 50 minutes). Drain, reserving ¼ cup cooking liquid.
2. Fit food processor with steel blade. Put carrot, shallots, and fresh herbs in workbowl. Process until carrots reach pinhead size. Add beans, spices, 2 tablespoons stock or reserved cooking liquid, Worcestershire sauce, oil, flour, and baking powder. Process in on/off turns until well combined but not a smooth purée. Scrape into bowl. Stir in ham and pepper. Chill for 20 minutes. Preheat oven to 350 degrees.
3. Sauté cakes in batches. Using pastry brush, spread a film of oil across nonstick skillet. Heat skillet until hot but not smoking. Drop spoonfuls of mixture into skillet, flattening with spatula to ¼-inch thickness. Sauté on each side until browned and crisp (about 4 minutes), regulating heat when successive batches are added. Keep cooked batches warm in preheated oven.
4. To serve as finger-food hors d'oeuvres, place each cake in center

of an arugula leaf. Sprinkle with lemon juice. Fold over leaves to form bundle. Secure with cocktail picks. Arrange on platter garnished with lemon wedges.

5. To serve the cakes as a first course, arrange arugula leaves across individual serving plates. Top with 2 or 3 cakes per plate, and garnish with lemon wedges and cucumber slices.

Yield: **About 15 cakes; serves 5 to 6**

EGGPLANT SHOESTRINGS

They're spicy, crunchy, and addictive!

2 tablespoons Italian olive oil
2 eggs (use 1 yolk and 2 whites)
1/4 cup evaporated skim milk
1 teaspoon mild curry powder
1/4 teaspoon freshly ground black
pepper
1 1 1/2-pound eggplant, scrubbed

and trimmed
3/4 cup Breading Mix (page 17)
2 tablespoons each red wine
vinegar and balsamic vinegar
2 teaspoons Worcestershire sauce
1/4 teaspoon salt (optional)

1. Position oven rack in lower section of oven. Preheat oven to 450 degrees. Spread oil across large rectangular metal pan (base measurement 10″ × 15″). Place pan in oven for 7 minutes.

2. In large bowl, combine eggs, milk, curry powder, and pepper. Beat with fork to blend.

3. Cut eggplant into 1/4-inch slices. Then cut slices crosswise into 1/4-inch strips. Immediately place in egg mixture, stirring to coat. Let stand for 2 minutes. Pour into colander and drain.

4. Spread half of the Breading Mix across a large sheet of wax paper. Place eggplant strips over mix. Strew remaining Breading Mix over all. Lift up sides of paper and shift mixture from side to side to coat evenly.

5. Take hot oiled pan from oven. Immediately strew eggplant across pan, separating pieces into one layer. Bake for 10 minutes. Scoop up and turn with spatula. Return to oven for 10 minutes.

6. In cup, combine vinegars. Sprinkle over strips, turning with spatula to combine. Return to oven for 5 minutes. Remove from oven. Drizzle with Worcestershire sauce. Taste for salt, adding a pinch if desired. Transfer to hot serving plate. Serve at once.

Yield: **Serves 6**

POLENTA APPETIZERS

An innovative way of serving polenta: Sauté shallots and peppers with a tinge of curry powder, combine with pimentos, a light cream cheese, and mustard, and spread atop warm seasoned polenta squares. Arrange the squares over watercress leaves (or radicchio cups) for an eye-catching presentation.

1 recipe Sautéed Polenta (page 62)

2 teaspoons Italian olive oil

1/3 cup each minced shallot and sweet green pepper

1 tablespoon minced garlic

1 1/2 teaspoons mild curry powder

1/2 teaspoon dried tarragon, crumbled

2 teaspoons red wine vinegar

2 tablespoons finely chopped and seeded ripe tomato

2 tablespoons minced parsley

3 whole unsalted pimentos, drained on paper toweling and chopped

3 tablespoons light cream cheese (Neufchâtel)

1 teaspoon each prepared Dijon mustard, preferably without salt, and fresh lemon juice

1 tablespoon Light Choice sour cream or plain low-fat yogurt

Watercress leaves or radicchio cups

1/4 teaspoon salt

Freshly ground black pepper

1. Prepare Sautéed Polenta recipe through Step 4. (Recipe may be prepared a day ahead and refrigerated.) Set aside.

2. Heat oil in small nonstick skillet. Add shallot, green pepper, and garlic. Sprinkle with curry powder and tarragon. Sauté over moderate heat until softened without browning (about 4 minutes). Combine vinegar with mixture. Stir in tomato and cook for 1 minute. Transfer to small bowl. Sprinkle with parsley.

3. On a flat dish, combine and mash all pimentos with cream cheese, mustard, and lemon juice. Add to bowl with sour cream or yogurt and mix.

4. Sauté polenta squares following directions in Step 5 of Sautéed Polenta recipe. Spread squares with equal amounts of prepared mixture. Arrange watercress leaves or radicchio cups on warmed plates and top with 2 or 3 polenta squares. Sprinkle with salt and pepper. Serve warm.

Yield: **Serves 4 to 6**

SWORDFISH NUGGETS

Meaty fresh swordfish is wonderful marinated in a mixture of tart lemon juice, slightly sweet full-bodied balsamic vinegar, and sharp Dijon mustard. Wrap chunks in a crisp envelope of Breading Mix, sauté quickly, and pierce with cocktail picks.

2 tablespoons fresh lemon juice
2 teaspoons Italian olive oil, plus
　　1 tablespoon
1 teaspoon balsamic vinegar
1/2 teaspoon dry mustard
1/4 teaspoon salt
2 tablespoons minced Italian flat
　　parsley
3/4 pound fresh swordfish, sliced

3/4-inch thick, cut into
3/4-inch chunks
4 to 5 tablespoons Breading Mix
　　(page 17)
1/8 to 1/4 teaspoon freshly ground
　　black pepper
2 tablespoons finely minced shallots
1/2 medium lemon
Lemon wedges

1. In medium bowl, whisk lemon juice, 2 teaspoons oil, vinegar, mustard, salt, and parsley. Add fish, turning several times to coat. Let stand, covered, at room temperature for 45 minutes. (Or refrigerate for several hours, returning to room temperature before proceeding with the next step.) Most of the marinade will be absorbed.
2. Combine Breading Mix with pepper. Sprinkle half across a sheet of wax paper. Drain fish and spread it over mix; sprinkle remaining mix over fish, rolling to coat evenly.
3. Heat remaining oil in a large nonstick skillet for 30 seconds. Strew with shallots. Cook, without stirring, for 30 seconds over medium-high heat. Arrange fish in skillet in a single layer without crowding (you may have to prepare two batches), and cook for 2 minutes without stirring. Turn. Cook for 2 more minutes. Repeat cooking and turning twice more until nuggets are crisp and brown (8 minutes total cooking time).
4. Sprinkle fish with lemon juice, pierce with cocktail picks, and serve on a warmed serving platter, garnished with lemon wedges.

Yield: **About 24 nuggets**

Serving suggestion: Serve with a dipping sauce on the side if desired. Barbecue Sauce (page 147) and Horseradish Sauce (page 152) are good accompaniments.

COCKTAIL CHICKEN CABOCHONS

"Cabochon" is a word jewelers use to describe a gem cut into a ball-like form. Here I've used the word to express the gemlike quality of these chicken balls.

2 large cloves garlic, peeled and
    halved
2 large shallots, peeled and
    quartered
3 teaspoons each Italian olive oil
    and sweet butter/margarine
    blend, combined
2 firmly packed cups cubed cooked
    chicken
2 teaspoons mild curry powder
1 teaspoon dried tarragon,
    crumbled
1/4 cup each fine bread crumbs
    (toasted) and toasted wheat

germ
1/8 teaspoon each salt and freshly
    ground white or black pepper
2 1/2 tablespoons freshly grated
    Parmesan cheese
1/4 cup each loosely packed parsley
    florets and fresh mint leaves,
    rinsed and well dried
1 tablespoon prepared white
    horseradish
3/4 cup dry sherry
1 small egg, lightly beaten
1/2 lemon

1. Fit workbowl of food processor with steel blade. With machine running, drop garlic and shallots through feed tube and process to fine-mince.
2. Heat 2 teaspoons oil in small nonstick skillet until hot. Scrape mixture from workbowl into skillet. Sauté over moderate heat until wilted but not brown. Return to workbowl. Add chicken, curry, tarragon, bread crumbs, wheat germ, salt, pepper, cheese, herbs, horseradish, 1/3 cup sherry, and egg. Process until well combined. Cover and chill in freezer for 15 minutes. Scoop up teaspoons of mixture and shape into 24 balls.
3. Heat remaining 4 teaspoons oil mix in large nonstick skillet until hot. Add balls, spreading across skillet. Sauté over medium-high heat, browning all over, gently shaking skillet from time to time. Pour remaining sherry around sides of skillet. Cook, without stirring, for 30 seconds. Combine balls with liquid and cook over medium-high heat, basting often, until all liquid is evaporated.
4. Sprinkle with lemon juice. Pierce with cocktail picks and serve hot.

Yield: **24 cocktail cabochons**

Variation: Serve as a pâté: Transfer processed mixture to covered dish and chill for 15 minutes. On individual serving plates, mound heaping tablespoons of mixture onto crisp lettuce cups or watercress leaves. Top with well-drained slivered unsalted pimentos. Serve with thin-sliced just-toasted French Bread (page 162) or Oat Crackers (page 155).

PIMENTO CREAM SAUCE TOPPING

Tastier, lower in fat, and far more versatile than sour cream topping, this herbed sauce doubles as a dip for vegetables, melba toast, or Oat Crackers (page 155). Try it, too, over steamed potatoes or chilled skinned tomato on a bed of crispy bitter-edged arugula.

½ cup low-fat ricotta cheese
½ cup Light Choice sour cream
¼ cup plain low-fat yogurt
½ teaspoon superfine sugar
2 teaspoons prepared unsalted
    Dijon mustard
2 teaspoons wine vinegar
2 tablespoons each minced parsley
    and fresh basil, mint, or dill

¼ cup minced scallion or onion
¼ teaspoon salt (optional)
¼ teaspoon freshly ground white
    or black pepper
4-ounce jar unsalted pimentos, well
    drained on paper toweling,
    minced
Cayenne pepper to taste

1. Put ricotta, sour cream, yogurt, sugar, and mustard in a small bowl. Stir briskly and blend. Then add vinegar, parsley, herbs, scallion, salt, pepper, pimentos, and cayenne, one at a time, stirring after each addition.
2. Transfer to jar. Cover and refrigerate for several hours or overnight so that flavors develop.

Yield: **Scant 2 cups**

SPICY PEANUT SPREAD

This is a versatile spread that is good on your morning toast, or with tea or cocktails. For ravenous kids, it's a good, satisfying, wholesome after-school snack that can beat the competition.

⅓ cup plain low-fat yogurt
⅓ cup unsalted dry-curd cottage cheese, or drained low-fat cottage cheese
3 tablespoons smooth unseasoned peanut butter
2 tablespoons Light Choice sour cream
⅛ teaspoon salt

¼ teaspoon each cinnamon and ground cardamom
1 tablespoon fresh lemon juice
1 tablespoon unhulled sesame seeds (available in health-food stores)
1 tablespoon unsweetened seedless jelly, such as blackberry or raspberry

1. Combine yogurt, cottage cheese, peanut butter, sour cream, salt, cinnamon, and lemon juice in blender. Blend on medium speed for 5 seconds. Scrape into bowl.
2. Stir in sesame seeds and jelly. Chill for at least 2 hours before serving (mixture will thicken). Serve with whole-grain crackers or toasted thin-sliced Masterpiece Bread (page 156).

Yield: **About 1¼ cups**

Notes:

1. When opening a fresh carton of dry-curd cottage cheese, mix thoroughly to incorporate skim milk liquid with solids.
2. If you use salted low-fat cottage cheese, eliminate the salt in the recipe.

FRUIT AND NUT CHEESE SPREAD

This appetizer can be used as a spread or a dip. It's good *with* soups and salads as well as *before* them.

3-inch piece orange zest from navel orange
1/4 cup coarsely chopped walnuts
1/4 cup firmly packed rinsed and dried parsley florets
1/2 cup low-fat cottage cheese
1/3 cup crushed unsweetened pineapple, well drained
1/2 teaspoon ground ginger

1/4 teaspoon cinnamon
2 teaspoons fresh lemon juice
1-inch piece lemon zest
1/8 teaspoon each salt and cayenne pepper
2 tablespoons Light Choice sour cream or plain low-fat yogurt (optional)

1. Mince orange zest by hand or in electric mini-chopper. Transfer to small plate and set aside.
2. Fit food processor with steel blade. Combine remaining ingredients in workbowl. In on/off turns, process mixture until well-chopped but not puréed. Scrape into bowl. Stir in sour cream or yogurt if desired. Chill.
3. Spread on flatbread crackers or thin-sliced bread triangles, and sprinkle with chopped orange zest. Or serve as a dip, piled into a small decorative bowl, sprinkled with orange zest. Celery and thin-sliced melba toast made from Masterpiece Bread (156) make sturdy dippers.

Yield: **About 1 1/4 cups**

5

VEGETABLES AND GRAINS

SKILLET "FRENCH-FRIED" POTATOES

Crispy, crunchy, brown, delicious. And guilt-free because they're not deep-fried! Here's a French-fried taste-alike you can enjoy often.

1 1/2 pounds Idaho or russet potatoes, peeled, cut into 1/4-inch strips
1 teaspoon each onion powder, mild curry powder, and dried

oregano leaves, crushed
2 tablespoons Italian olive oil
Dash of Worcestershire sauce
1/4 teaspoon salt (optional)

1. Soak potatoes in ice water for 30 minutes. Drain on paper toweling; dry completely.
2. In cup combine onion powder, curry powder, and oregano. Set aside.
3. Spread half the oil across each of two well-seasoned iron skillets (or all the oil in one large iron griddle) and heat until very hot but not smoking. Spread potatoes across skillet in one layer. Over medium-high heat, cook without stirring for 3 minutes. Carefully scoop up and turn with spatula. Sprinkle evenly with seasoning mix. Continue cooking and turning, regulating heat when necessary, until potatoes are tender and browned all over (about 15 minutes).
4. Sprinkle with Worcestershire sauce (don't use too much or potatoes will become soggy), and continue cooking for 30 seconds. Sprinkle with salt, and toss. Serve at once on warm uncovered serving dish.

Yield: **Serves 4**

CRISPY OVEN-BAKED POTATO PANCAKES

With less moisture than most potatoes, the Idaho is just perfect for this new way of creating *crispy* potato pancakes. Serve them as a side dish or as a base for sautéed or broiled meats, fish, or poultry, or even as a sauce-napped lid for fish or seafood. They'll absorb the flavors of the foods they accompany while asserting their own character, as all great potato pancakes should.

1 1/2 pounds Idaho potatoes, peeled
1 teaspoon each mild curry powder and dried crushed oregano
1/2 teaspoon chili con carne seasoning or chili powder
1/4 teaspoon salt
1/8 teaspoon freshly ground white
or black pepper
2 tablespoons minced shallot
2 tablespoons unbleached flour
3 teaspoons Italian olive oil
Rice vinegar or Worcestershire sauce

1. Preheat oven to 500 degrees. Grate potatoes coarsely by hand or julienne with food processor. If using processor, fit bowl with grating attachment. Cut each potato in half, and then each half into lengthwise thirds. Standing them upright, push them through feed tube with gentle pressure. Turn into colander; rinse under cold water for 10 seconds. Invert colander onto clean absorbent dishcloth or doubled paper toweling, pressing out as much moisture as possible. Place in bowl.
2. In cup, combine seasonings, shallot, and flour. Work mixture into potatoes with fingers to distribute evenly. Chill for 15 minutes.
3. Set out 2 cookie sheets. Using scrunched-up piece of wax paper, rub 1 1/2 teaspoons oil across each sheet. Compress potatoes with hands. Arrange 4 mounds on each cookie sheet, pressing to 5-inch circles, each 1/4 inch thick, leaving no spaces within each pancake.
4. Bake for 12 to 15 minutes, pressing each pancake down with spatula after 10 minutes. Loosen around each pancake and carefully flip over. Return to oven and bake until crisp (5 to 6 minutes). Serve on a warm platter, sprinkling on vinegar or Worcestershire sauce to taste.

Yield: **8 pancakes**

Variation: Substitute 1 tablespoon Savory Seasoning (page 15) for curry powder, oregano, and chili seasonings, and add 2 tablespoons peeled and finely grated carrot in Step 2.

ZESTY SMOOTH POTATOES

A departure from the same old mashed potatoes. Curry, tomato paste, and garlic cloves give them an exotic twist. Baked in a hot oven, the once prosaic potato emerges puffed up almost like a soufflé.

1 1/2 pounds Idaho or russet potatoes, peeled and cut into 1/2-inch cubes
6 large cloves garlic, peeled and halved
3 teaspoons sweet butter/margarine blend
2 teaspoons mild curry powder
1/8 teaspoon salt
3 tablespoons Parmesan cheese

1 tablespoon unsalted tomato paste
1/8 teaspoon cayenne pepper
2 tablespoons each plain low-fat yogurt and Light Choice sour cream, or 4 tablespoons yogurt
2 tablespoons milk
2 tablespoons minced fresh parsley or basil
Dash of paprika

1. Put potatoes and garlic in heavy-bottomed 2-quart saucepan. Cover with water and bring to rolling boil. Reduce to a slow boil and cook until potatoes are tender and still flaky (12 to 15 minutes). Drain in colander. Return to saucepan and cook for 30 seconds over moderate heat until all moisture evaporates. Put through ricer or food mill, then into a bowl. Stir in 2 teaspoons shortening.
2. Preheat oven to 400 degrees.
3. Sprinkle potato mixture with curry, salt, and 2 tablespoons Parmesan and blend. In a cup, mix tomato paste with cayenne pepper, yogurt, sour cream, and milk. Combine with potatoes. Stir in parsley or basil.
4. Pile mixture into a 7-inch lightly greased soufflé dish or ovenproof crock. Sprinkle with remaining 1 tablespoon Parmesan; cut remaining 1 teaspoon shortening into small pieces and dot pieces over mixture. Top with several dashes of paprika and bake until heated through (10 to 12 minutes).

Yield: **Serves 4 to 5**

WHITE SWEET POTATOES WITH PIMENTOS

White sweet potatoes (also called white sweets) have a lemony tint, and are faintly sweet. They are more finely textured than yams, less moist, and when prepared my way come to the table silky-smooth, a delectable accompaniment to meat and poultry.

3 medium white sweet potatoes (about 1 3/4 pounds), cut into 1-inch cubes
1/4 teaspoon cinnamon
1/2 teaspoon mild curry powder
1/4 teaspoon salt
5 teaspoons Italian olive oil
1/4 cup minced onion or scallion

2 tablespoons frozen orange juice concentrate
1/4 cup plain low-fat yogurt
3 tablespoons rinsed, dried, and minced fresh coriander
3 tablespoons minced and well-drained unsalted pimentos

1. Put potatoes in large heavy-bottomed saucepan. Cover with water and boil until tender but not oversoft. Drain in colander. Return potatoes to saucepan and cook over medium-high heat about 30 seconds, shaking pan, until all liquid evaporates. Remove from heat and mash with cinnamon, curry powder, and half the salt.
2. Heat 1 teaspoon oil in small nonstick skillet until hot. Add onion or scallion and sauté for 2 minutes over moderate heat, taking care not to brown. Add to potatoes with remaining oil.
3. In a cup, combine orange juice concentrate with yogurt. Stir into potatoes, then gently fold in coriander and pimentos. Add remaining half of salt if desired.
4. Reheat just before serving and transfer to warm serving bowl, or pile into 4 lightly oiled ovenproof custard-size crocks and bake in preheated 425-degree oven until heated through and lightly browned.

Yield: **Serves 4**

Note: To prevent white sweets from darkening after cutting, drop immediately into a bowl of cold water.

TOFU POTATO PANCAKES

Here I take advantage of tofu's moist texture to create a potato pancake that's soft on the inside and crisp on the outside. Parmesan cheese and a hint of whole wheat flour enhance the far-from-traditional flavor.

*1 medium Idaho potato (¹/₂
    pound), cut into ¹/₂-inch
    cubes
1 cup drained, dried, and mashed
    tofu
3 tablespoons freshly grated
    Parmesan cheese
1 tablespoon fresh lemon juice
¹/₂ cup finely minced onion
¹/₄ teaspoon each cinnamon and*

*freshly grated nutmeg
¹/₂ teaspoon mild curry powder
3 tablespoons stone-ground whole
    wheat flour
2 tablespoons minced parsley or
    coriander
1 small egg, well beaten with fork
2 teaspoons each Italian olive oil
    and sweet butter/margarine
    blend*

1. Cook potato in boiling water to cover until pieces are tender but not frayed at the edges (about 12 minutes). Drain in colander and return to saucepan. Cook briefly over medium-high heat until all moisture evaporates (about 30 seconds). Transfer to bowl and mash.
2. Add tofu and Parmesan, and mash ingredients until well blended. Stir in lemon juice and onion.
3. Combine spices with flour. Sprinkle over mixture. Add parsley or coriander and blend. Pour in egg and beat with wooden spoon. Cover and place in freezer for 20 minutes. Divide into 16 parts. Shape into balls.
4. Preheat oven (or tabletop oven/toaster) to 350 degrees.
5. Using large nonstick skillet, cook pancakes in 4 batches. Heat ¹/₂ teaspoon each oil and shortening in skillet until hot, tilting pan to distribute evenly. Arrange 4 balls in skillet, flattening gently with spatula to ³/₈ inch. Sauté over medium-high heat on each side until browned. Transfer to plate and keep warm in oven. Repeat procedure for remaining pancakes.

Yield: 16 pancakes; serves 4 as a main course

Variation: Substitute 1 ¹/₂ teaspoons Savory Seasoning (page 15) for spices listed.

Serving suggestion: Sherried Applesauce (page 206) goes nicely with these pancakes, either as a topping or a side dish.

POTATO AND APPLE MEDLEY

I've mixed yams (with their dense sweetness) with white sweet potatoes (which are faintly sweet) and Idahos (bland and flaky)—and added a Golden Delicious apple. Result: a purée that's a perfect foil for poultry or roasted meat.

1 each Idaho potato, white sweet potato, and yam (1 3/4 to 2 pounds), cut into 1/2-inch cubes
1 small Golden Delicious apple, cored, peeled, and cut into 1-inch cubes
3/4 teaspoon each ground coriander, cinnamon, and dried tarragon leaves

1/4 teaspoon salt
4 teaspoons sweet butter/margarine blend
2 tablespoons minced shallot
2 tablespoons dry sherry
2 tablespoons coarsely chopped parsley or fresh mint, or a combination of both
2 tablespoons Light Choice sour cream or plain low-fat yogurt

1. Cook potatoes in a large saucepan of briskly boiling water to cover until almost tender (about 11 minutes). Add apple and continue boiling, stirring from time to time, until potatoes are firm-tender. Drain in colander. Return to saucepan and over moderate heat, turn with large spoon to remove excess moisture.
2. Remove saucepan from heat. Stir in seasonings and shortening. Put through ricer or mash (do not use food processor). Stir in shallot; blend in sherry. Add herb(s) and fold in sour cream or yogurt.
3. Reheat briefly, taking care that mixture doesn't stick to pan. Turn into a warm serving bowl and serve piping hot. (This mixture may also be piled into a 7-inch lightly greased soufflé dish and baked in a preheated 400-degree oven until heated through, about 20 minutes).

Yield: **Serves 6**

THREE-PEPPER SAUTÉ

A colorful melange for that very special occasion when your palate craves something new. It is a good complement for simply grilled fish, chicken, or meat.

1 large sweet red pepper
1 large sweet green pepper
1 large sweet yellow pepper
2 teaspoons unhulled sesame seeds
   (available in health-food
   stores)
1/2 ounce dried shiitake mushrooms
2 teaspoons unseasoned Oriental

sesame oil
1 tablespoon each minced ginger
   and garlic
1/2 cup crisp watercress leaves
1 1/2 teaspoons low-sodium soy
   sauce
1/4 teaspoon salt (optional)

1. Char peppers following Step 1 in the recipe for Saffron Rice (page 174). After final rinsing, cut into 1/4-inch strips and drain on paper toweling.
2. Strew sesame seeds across hot skillet or wok. Toast over medium-high heat, shaking pan from side to side, until seeds begin to pop. Transfer to cup.
3. Break up mushrooms. Place in colander and rinse under cold running water. Transfer to cup. Add enough boiling water to barely cover. Let soak for 20 minutes. Squeeze out, reserving liquid, and chop coarsely.
4. Heat oil in wok or large nonstick skillet until hot. Add ginger and garlic. Sauté over medium-high heat for 30 seconds. Stir in peppers and sauté for 1 minute more. Add mushrooms and watercress; sauté for 1 minute. Add reserved mushroom liquid and soy sauce. Sauté over high heat for 30 seconds. Season with salt if desired.
5. Arrange mixture in heated bowl. Sprinkle with toasted sesame seeds and serve hot.

Yield: **Serves 4**

GREEN BEAN AND BOK CHOY SAUTÉ

For super-crunch texture, prepare in a wok; for a more tender rendition, use a nonstick skillet.

½ pound fresh tender young green beans, julienned

2 tablespoons blanched almonds

2 teaspoons peanut oil or Italian olive oil

1 tablespoon Vegetable Mix (page 18)

2 cups ½-inch slices fresh bok choy, including some of the

leaves (about 1 small bunch)

¼ teaspoon cumin

½ teaspoon mild curry powder

⅛ teaspoon salt

2 whole unsalted pimentos, drained, cut into strips

1 tablespoon dry sherry

2 tablespoons coarsely chopped well-rinsed fresh coriander

1. Steam green beans for 8 minutes. Rinse under cold running water. Set aside.

2. Heat a small nonstick skillet. Strew with almonds and toast lightly. (Steps 1 and 2 may be prepared well in advance of cooking time.)

3. Spread oil across wok or large nonstick skillet. Heat until hot but not smoking. Add Vegetable Mix, and stir-fry (cook and stir) for 30 seconds. Add bok choy. Sprinkle with seasonings. Stir-fry over medium-high heat for 2 minutes. Stir in green beans.

4. Add pimentos, separating strips. Pour sherry around sides of wok or skillet. Combine with mixture and cook for 1 minute. Sprinkle in nuts. Remove from heat and top with coriander. Serve immediately.

Yield: **Serves 4**

SAUTÉED ZUCCHINI WITH HORSERADISH

Zucchini undergoes an instant personality change when sparked with sharp horseradish and curry. I temper the spiciness with dollops of light sour cream and yogurt.

1 1/2 tablespoons Italian olive oil
2 tablespoons Vegetable Mix (page 18)
3 medium zucchini, well scrubbed, cut into 1/2-inch cubes
1 large onion, coarsely chopped
1 1/2 teaspoons each mild curry powder and dried tarragon, crumbled
1/4 pound snow-white fresh

mushrooms, ends trimmed, damp-wiped, and thin-sliced
1 1/2 tablespoons prepared white horseradish
3 tablespoons Light Choice sour cream
1 tablespoon plain low-fat yogurt
1/8 teaspoon each salt and freshly grated ground white pepper

1. Heat oil in large nonstick skillet until hot. Add Vegetable Mix. Sauté over medium heat for 30 seconds. Add zucchini and onion and sauté for 2 minutes.
2. Sprinkle in curry and tarragon. Stir in mushrooms. Sauté all ingredients until zucchini is softened but still firm (about 6 minutes). Remove from heat.
3. Combine horseradish with sour cream or yogurt. Fold into vegetables with salt. Return to stove briefly to reheat, taking care not to boil.
4. Transfer to warm serving bowl and sprinkle with pepper. Serve very hot.

Yield: **Serves 4**

CARROT/CAULIFLOWER PURÉE

Combined with sweet carrots and tempered with yogurt and low-fat sour cream, cauliflower emerges as a star at the dinner table.

1 small head cauliflower, broken into florets (about 2 cups)
3 large carrots, peeled and trimmed, cut into ½-inch rounds
1 tablespoon sweet butter/margarine blend
2 large cloves garlic, coarsely chopped
½ teaspoon ground cardamom
¼ teaspoon salt
⅛ teaspoon cayenne pepper
6 sprigs parsley, florets only
2 tablespoons plain low-fat yogurt
1 tablespoon Light Choice sour cream

1. Steam cauliflower and carrot until crisp-tender. Place in workbowl of food processor fitted with steel blade.
2. Heat shortening in small nonstick skillet. Strew garlic across skillet. Sprinkle in cardamom, salt, and cayenne pepper. Combine and sauté until garlic is tender but not brown. Add to workbowl. Drop in parsley florets. Process until puréed and smooth. Pour into top of double boiler and reheat slowly.
3. Blend in yogurt and sour cream 1 minute before serving, warming briefly while stirring. Spoon into warmed serving dish and serve at once.

Yield: **Serves 4**

LIGHT CORN PUDDING

One of the most delicate-tasting puddings you will ever have. Serve it with broiled fish, meat, or poultry, or as a satisfying luncheon accompanied by a crisp green salad.

2 cups cut corn, fresh or frozen
³/₄ cup each skim milk and whole milk
¹/₄ teaspoon salt
¹/₈ teaspoon white or black pepper
¹/₂ teaspoon dried dill weed
2 teaspoons Savory Seasoning (page 15)
1 tablespoon each Italian olive oil and sweet butter/margarine blend
1 medium-size sweet red pepper, seeded, coarsely chopped

1 medium-size onion, coarsely chopped
1 tablespoon coarsely chopped garlic
3 eggs, separated (use 1 yolk and 3 whites)
2 tablespoons light cream or milk
2 tablespoons freshly grated Parmesan cheese
2 tablespoons unbleached flour
2 tablespoons minced fresh coriander or parsley

1. Preheat oven to 350 degrees. In medium-size heavy-bottomed saucepan, combine first six ingredients. Bring to boil. Reduce heat to simmering and cook, uncovered, for 8 minutes; avoid scorching. Remove mixture from stove and let cool. Pour into workbowl of food processor that has been fitted with steel blade. Process until corn is coarsely chopped (10 to 12 seconds). Scrape into bowl.
2. Heat oil and shortening in small nonstick skillet. Over medium heat, sauté red pepper, onion, and garlic until limp. Add to corn mixture.
3. In cup, beat egg yolk and cream or milk with fork to blend, then stir in cheese, flour, and coriander or parsley.
4. Beat egg whites until stiff peaks form. Quickly fold into pudding. Pour into lightly greased 2-quart baking dish. Bake, uncovered, in lower section of oven until lightly browned and puffed up (35 to 40 minutes). Serve immediately. Puff will recede slightly after spooning first serving.

Yield: **Serves 5 to 6**

QUINOA PILAF

Quinoa (pronounced *Keen-wa*), touted as "the supergrain of the future," was indeed a supergrain of the past among the ancient Incas, perhaps because of its protein content, which is higher than that of any other grain. It has a flavor all its own that makes it a refreshing alternate to more familiar grains. Quinoa is available in some supermarkets, in gourmet groceries, and in health-food stores.

2 cups Vegetable or Chicken Stock (pages 20, 19), or 1 cup each stock and water
⅔ cup Quinoa
½ teaspoon ground cumin
¼ teaspoon salt
1 teaspoon dried rosemary, crushed
1 tablespoon Italian olive oil
1 small sweet red pepper, seeded and coarsely chopped
½ cup coarsely chopped onion or scallion
2 teaspoons minced garlic
¼ pound snow-white fresh mushrooms, damp-wiped and sliced
2 tablespoons each coarsely chopped parsley and fresh coriander
1 tablespoon sweet butter/margarine blend
1½ teaspoons prepared Dijon mustard
1¼ cups unsalted chopped canned Italian plum tomatoes
¼ cup freshly grated Parmesan cheese
Pinch cayenne pepper

1. Place stock in medium-size heavy-bottomed saucepan. Bring to rolling boil. Add Quinoa, cumin, salt, and rosemary. Stir. Reduce heat to simmering. Cover tightly and simmer for 12 to 15 minutes, stirring 3 times at equal intervals. Liquid should be completely absorbed. Set aside.
2. Preheat oven to 400 degrees.
3. Heat oil in nonstick skillet over medium heat. Sauté pepper, onion, garlic, and mushrooms until very lightly browned (about 4 minutes), stirring continuously. Combine mixture with cooked Quinoa. Stir in parsley, coriander, and sweet butter/margarine blend. Blend mustard with tomatoes and gently stir into pilaf. Fold in cheese and cayenne pepper.
4. Spoon pilaf into a lightly greased 1¾-quart decorative ovenproof casserole. Cover and bake in center section of oven for 15 minutes. Uncover and bake for 10 more minutes. Serve directly from casserole.

Yield: **Serves 4 to 5**

MADEIRA DUXELLES

No matter when in a meal I serve this dish it disappears like lightning. I serve it as a first course spooned over thin-sliced cucumbers surrounded by slivered roast peppers. I serve it as a spread on toasted French bread, as an accompaniment to clear broths. I serve it as a taste-enhancer in some recipes. A double recipe might just be in order!

*2 large shallots, peeled and
    quartered*
*1 large clove garlic, peeled and
    halved*
1 dime-size-slice fresh ginger, peeled
*1 pound snow-white fresh
    mushrooms, ends trimmed,
    damp-wiped, quartered*

Florets from 4 large sprigs parsley
*2 teaspoons each sweet
    butter/margarine blend and
    Italian olive oil*
*1/2 teaspoon each mild curry
    powder and dried oregano*
1/4 teaspoon salt (optional)
1/3 cup Malmsey Madeira

1. Fit food processor with steel blade. Set workbowl on base. With machine running, drop shallots, garlic, and ginger through feed tube. Process until finely minced. Scrape onto plate.
2. Add mushrooms and parsley to workbowl. Process for 5 seconds. Scrape down sides of bowl. Process on/off several times until mushrooms reach the size of pinheads. (It's best to stop the processor and check mushrooms after 2 on/off turns.)
3. Heat shortening and oil in large nonstick skillet. Over moderate heat, sauté shallot mix for 1 minute. Then add mushrooms, sprinkle with seasonings, and cook for 5 minutes, stirring often. Mushrooms will give up some of their juices. Continue cooking while stirring until all liquid evaporates.
4. Stir in 1 tablespoon of wine at a time, letting it evaporate before adding the next tablespoon. After 20 minutes, duxelles will be fully cooked and take on a deep mahogany hue.
5. Refrigerate in a jar for use within 4 days, or pile into plastic container(s) and freeze.

Yield: **A little more than 1 cup**

Variation: Substitute 2 teaspoons Savory Seasoning (page 15) for oregano, curry powder, and salt.

Note: Frozen duxelles are easily broken up with a sharp knife should you need a tablespoon or two. Defrost before adding to your sauté pan.

EIGHT-MINUTE KASHA

Kasha translates from the Russian as coarse, cracked buckwheat seeds or buckwheat groats. Buckwheat is not a wheat at all, but an herb, almost like wheat nutritionally, with a distinctive flavor that's made it a favorite in Eastern Europe.

But there it's prepared as a sort of mush. Follow the instructions on packages of American kasha, and that's just what you'll get. I've developed a way to cook kasha so that the groats are fluffy and nut-textured, bringing out this unusual grain's full flavor.

This is a basic recipe you can use to spin off on your own. And it makes a good choice when you tire of rice and potatoes.

1 tablespoon Italian olive oil
2 tablespoons minced shallot
1 cup whole kasha (see Note*)*
About 2½ cups Vegetable or
*   Chicken Stock (pages 20,*
*   19), warmed*
1 tablespoon Savory Seasoning

(page 15)
1½ teaspoons white wine
*   Worcestershire sauce*
⅛ to ¼ teaspoon salt
2 teaspoons sweet butter/margarine
*   blend*
3 tablespoons minced chives

1. In heavy-bottomed 2-quart saucepan, heat oil until moderately hot. Add shallot. Sauté over medium heat for 30 seconds. Add kasha and cook for 2 minutes, stirring often.
2. Add 2¼ cups stock, Savory Seasoning, and Worcestershire sauce. Bring to boil. Reduce heat to a slow boil (a little hotter than simmering). Cook, uncovered, for 8 minutes, stirring often, particularly toward end of cooking time, adding remaining ¼ cup stock if liquid evaporates too rapidly. All liquid should be absorbed and kernels should be tender but not oversoft. Remove from heat.
3. Sprinkle in half the salt, shortening, and chives. Add the remaining salt if desired. Cover and let stand for 3 minutes. Fluff up and serve at once.

Yield: **Serves 4 to 5**

Variations:

1. Add 2 tablespoons freshly grated Parmesan cheese at the end of Step 3.
2. Substitute coarsely chopped fresh basil, rosemary, tarragon, or coriander for chives. The fresh herbs contribute to the bright taste.

3. Add 2 damp-wiped coarsely chopped snow-white fresh mushrooms and combine with shallots in Step 1.

Note: Kasha is sold in medium, small, and whole granulation. I prefer the hardier whole granulation.

COUSCOUS WITH FRUIT AND VEGETABLES

Let's not get into a hassle about which is better—uncooked or precooked couscous. I'm going with precooked. It's available in the supermarket. I can prepare it rapidly. And it's a tasty accessory for simply cooked meats, poultry, and vegetables. You may find, as I have, that precooked couscous makes an exciting addition to your list of kitchen staples.

2 teaspoons Italian olive oil
2 tablespoons minced shallot
2 large snow-white fresh
mushrooms, trimmed,
damp-wiped, and coarsely
chopped
3/4 cup precooked couscous
1 cup Chicken or Vegetable Stock
(pages 19, 20)
1/4 cup fresh orange juice

1/4 cup Malmsey Madeira
2 teaspoons Savory Seasoning
(page 15)
1/4 cup raisins or chopped dried
dates
2 tablespoons finely grated carrot
2 tablespoons coarsely chopped
Italian flat parsley
2 teaspoons sweet butter/margarine
blend

1. Heat oil in medium heavy-bottomed saucepan until hot. Over medium-high heat, sauté shallot and mushrooms until lightly browned, stirring constantly. Add couscous, stir well, and cook for 1 minute.
2. Add all remaining ingredients except shortening. Bring to a boil. Remove from heat, stir, and cover. Let stand for 7 minutes. Mix in shortening. Fluff up with a fork and serve at once.

Yield: **Serves 4 to 5**

SAUTÉED POLENTA

Polenta, a favorite in northern Italy, often takes the place of potatoes and stuffings on my gourmet menus. Prepare it ahead of time, then seven minutes before serving, sauté it with shallots and sprinkle with fresh herbs. It also makes a delightful appetizer (see page 40).

2 1/2 cups boiling water
1 cup Chicken or Vegetable Stock
    (pages 19, 20)
1 cup stone-ground yellow
    cornmeal
3 tablespoons minced shallot
1 tablespoon Savory Seasoning
    (page 15)

1/4 cup freshly grated Parmesan
    cheese
2 tablespoons sweet
    butter/margarine blend
1 tablespoon Italian olive oil
Minced fresh herbs such as
    coriander, rosemary, parsley,
    or dill

1. Pour 1 cup boiling water into a small bowl. Stir in 1/2 cup stock. Whisk in cornmeal until well blended.
2. Bring remaining water and stock to boil. Add 1 tablespoon shallot and seasoning. Boil for 1 minute. Then slowly, while whisking, add cornmeal mixture. Cook on low heat, uncovered, whisking often, for 10 minutes.
3. Again using whisk, blend Parmesan into mixture. Cook until very thick and smooth, adjusting heat when necessary to prevent scorching (about 20 minutes). Stir in 1 tablespoon shortening.
4. Lightly grease a 9-inch-square pan with shortening. Spread mixture evenly into pan. Let cool for 10 minutes. Cover and let stand until completely cooled. Cut into 12 squares. (May be covered and refrigerated up to this point until ready to use.)
5. Prepare squares in 2 batches in large nonstick skillet, using half the remaining shortening and oil, and half of the minced shallot for each batch. Heat the shortening and oil in skillet, spread with shallot, and cook for 30 seconds. Arrange polenta over shallot. Over medium heat, sauté on each side until light brown (3 to 4 minutes). Transfer to a warm serving plate and cover with sheet of wax paper. Sauté second batch. Sprinkle with minced fresh herbs of your choice and serve.

Yield: **Serves 4**

Variation: For a luncheon main course, sauté (Step 5), top with Tomato Sauce (p. 23) and sprinkle with freshly grated Parmesan cheese.

WILD RICE AND BARLEY MEDLEY

This exotic dish pairs a grass seed with a cereal seed. The grass seed is wild rice (not a rice at all, actually) and the cereal seed is barley.

½ cup wild rice, rinsed
¼ cup pearl barley, rinsed
1 ½ cups water
1 cup Vegetable Stock (page 20)
1 teaspoon each mild curry powder
  and dried oregano
¼ teaspoon each ground ginger
  and salt
2 large snow-white fresh

mushrooms, ends trimmed,
  damp-wiped, coarsely chopped
1 ½ tablespoons each finely minced
  fresh coriander and Italian
  flat parsley
1 teaspoon Worcestershire sauce
½ cup just-cooked fresh peas
2 tablespoons freshly grated
  Parmesan cheese

1. In 1¾- to 2-quart heavy-bottomed saucepan, combine rice, barley, water, stock, and seasonings, stirring several times. Let soak for 2 hours.
2. Bring mixture to boil. Add mushrooms, 2 tablespoons coriander or parsley, and Worcestershire sauce. Reduce heat to low. Cover and simmer until all liquid is absorbed (about 40 minutes). Stir in peas.
3. Sprinkle in cheese and remaining coriander or parsley, gently combining. Cover and let stand for 3 minutes before serving.

Yield: **Serves 4**

PASTA WITH ONION/SHALLOT SAUCE

Welcome a new pasta sauce with three different tastes! Onions, shallot, and ginger are slow-cooked with wine until golden. Then rich stock, seasonings, and a small amount of light cream is added to make a subtly sweet sauce. If the pasta is served with fish, use Fish Stock; with meat or poultry, Chicken Stock; and with vegetables, Vegetable Stock. Three different sauces—three different tastes.

2 1/2 tablespoons Italian olive oil
4 1/2 cups thinly sliced onion
  (about 1 pound)
1/4 cup coarsely chopped shallot
1 teaspoon minced fresh ginger
1/4 teaspoon dried thyme leaves,
  crushed
2/3 cup dry white wine
1/2 pound snow-white fresh
  mushrooms, ends trimmed,
  damp-wiped, quartered, and
  thinly sliced

1/8 teaspoon salt
1/2 cup Fish, Chicken, or Vegetable
  Stock (pages 19–21)
3 tablespoons light cream
3 tablespoons minced parsley
4 tablespoons freshly grated
  Parmesan cheese
1/2 teaspoon freshly grated nutmeg
1/4 teaspoon freshly ground black
  or white pepper
6 ounces capellini

1. In large heavy-bottomed saucepan, heat 1 tablespoon oil. Add onion, shallots, ginger, and thyme. Stir and cook over moderate heat for 3 minutes. Add 1/3 cup wine, cover, and cook for 20 minutes, stirring twice at equal intervals, and lowering heat when necessary to prevent onions from sticking to saucepan. Reduce heat to low. Continue cooking for 20 minutes longer, stirring from time to time as onion mix begins to turn golden brown.
2. While sauce cooks, heat remaining 1 1/2 tablespoons oil in large nonstick skillet. Sauté mushrooms over moderate heat for 2 minutes. Sprinkle with salt. Sauté for 1 minute longer. Remove from heat and set aside.
3. After onions have finished cooking, stir in remaining 1/3 cup wine. Place saucepan over moderately high heat for 1 minute. Stir in stock and cook for 1 minute. Then add cream, 2 tablespoons parsley, 3 tablespoons Parmesan cheese, nutmeg, and pepper. Combine and cook for 30 seconds. Stir in mushrooms. Cover. Remove from heat.

4. Bring pot of water to rolling boil. Add capellini (it cooks within 3 minutes). Drain thoroughly in colander. Add to sauce, stirring to combine. Reheat briefly. Serve in warm bowl, sprinkled with remaining 1 tablespoon parsley and 1 tablespoon Parmesan.

Yield: **Serves 4 to 5 as a main course**

CREPES

Use these thin, delectable pancakes as attractive envelopes for seafood, vegetables, or cheese. They're remarkably easy to make and they freeze well. For another exciting culinary experience, see Shrimp-Filled Crepes (page 106).

¼ cup each cake flour (not self-rising) and unbleached flour
⅛ teaspoon salt
2 large eggs (use 1 yolk and 2 whites)

1 tablespoon dry sherry or Madeira
¼ cup each skim and whole milk, or ½ cup whole milk
2 tablespoons plus 2 teaspoons melted sweet butter/margarine blend

1. Sift flours and salt into medium bowl. In cup, lightly beat eggs and sherry with fork. Whisk into flour mixture. Gradually add milk and whisk until very smooth. Stir in 2 tablespoons shortening. Let stand for 30 minutes. Stir gently before using.
2. Place 8-inch nonstick omelet pan over moderate heat. Using pastry brush, lightly coat with shortening. Heat until a drop of water dropped in bounces off. Ladle in 2½ tablespoons batter, immediately tilting skillet to evenly distribute across pan. Cook until set and lightly brown (about 2 minutes). Lift up sides, turn, and cook for 30 seconds. Repeat procedure, regulating heat from time to time and stacking crepes, second side up, as they're made.

Yield: **10 to 11 crepes**

BUCKWHEAT SPÄTZLE

The popular German noodle dish, spätzle, traditionally a very heavy food, is presented here in a light version. It's so flavorful (buckwheat is the secret) that you can even do without the high-calorie gravy that usually supplies the moisture and taste.

2 large eggs
1/2 cup whole milk
1/4 cup water
1/4 teaspoon salt
1 1/4 cups unbleached flour
1/4 cup buckwheat flour
1/4 teaspoon each ground cardamom and freshly grated nutmeg
1 1/2 tablespoons sweet

butter/margarine blend
3 tablespoons minced shallot, or 2 tablespoons Vegetable Mix (page 18)
2 tablespoons freshly grated Parmesan cheese
1/4 cup loosely packed fresh basil leaves
Freshly ground black or white pepper

1. Break eggs into large bowl and whisk with milk, water, and half the salt until well blended. Sift flours and spices into mixture. Stir with wooden spoon (do not whisk) until dry ingredients are incorporated and mixture is smooth and thick.
2. Bring large pot of water to boil. Add remaining 1/8 teaspoon salt. Place 1/4-inch-holed colander over boiling water. Pour batter into colander. Stir mixture with wooden spoon so spätzle drips through holes. It will immediately jell and puff up into irregularly shaped noodles and rise to the top. Reduce heat and slow-boil for 1 minute. Pour contents of pot into strainer. Place under gently running cold water, then drain completely. (Recipe may be prepared an hour ahead of time up to this point, covered, and refrigerated.)
3. Heat shortening in large nonstick skillet until hot. Add shallot or vegetable mix. Sauté over medium heat for 30 seconds; spread across skillet. Add spätzle and gently sauté until heated through, stirring several times. Sprinkle in Parmesan and basil, stirring briefly. Turn into warmed serving bowl and sprinkle with pepper.

Yield: **Serves 4 to 5**

Variation: A combination of scant 1/4 cup coarsely chopped fresh mint and 1 tablespoon minced parsley may be substituted for basil.

Note: Buckwheat flour is available in most health-food stores.

6
CHICKEN

CHICKEN IN TOMATO SAUCE

This chicken is dredged in a light coating, browned, then simmered in my Tomato Sauce until tangy and tender.

4 teaspoons cornstarch
1 teaspoon mild curry powder
1 3- to 3 1/2-pound broiling
  chicken, skinned, cut into
  eighths
1 1/2 tablespoons Italian olive oil
2 tablespoons balsamic vinegar

1 1/4 cups Tomato Sauce (page 23)
4 sprigs dill, tied into neat bundle
  with white cotton thread
1 teaspoon caraway seed, partially
  crushed
2 tablespoons fresh lemon juice
1/8 to 1/4 teaspoon salt

1. In a cup, combine cornstarch and curry powder, stirring to blend. Sprinkle across large sheet of wax paper. Pierce chicken pieces all over with sharp-pronged fork. Dredge in mixture, first pressing each side to adhere, then shaking off excess.

2. Heat oil in large well-seasoned iron skillet until hot. Over medium-high heat, brown chicken on each side for 3 minutes, scooping up with spatula to turn and adjusting heat when necessary to prevent scorching. Transfer to a plate.

3. Keeping your head back from the stove, pour in vinegar (it will smoke up for a moment). Scrape skillet to loosen any cracklings. Cook for a few seconds. Add Tomato Sauce and bring to a boil. Drop in dill bundle and caraway seeds. Return browned chicken to skillet, turning several times to coat. Bring liquid to a simmering point. Cover tightly and cook for 45 to 50 minutes, or until tender, turning and spooning with sauce 3 times at equal intervals. Dribble in lemon juice; sprinkle with salt. Spoon sauce all over chicken pieces, cover, and remove from heat. Let stand for 15 minutes.

4. Transfer chicken with slotted spoon to warm serving plate; cover to keep warm. Discard dill bundle after pressing out juices. Raise heat under skillet to medium-high, and reduce sauce by half. Ladle over chicken and serve at once.

Yield: **Serves 4**

CHICKEN WITH SAFFRON-TOMATO SAUCE

Minimum fuss, minimum ingredients, maximum enjoyment. A striking presentation that tastes like it took extensive preparation. But it's yours, from start to finish, in only 45 minutes!

1 1/2 tablespoons Italian olive oil
1 tablespoon minced garlic
1/2 cup coarsely chopped onion
1 medium sweet green pepper,
*   seeded, cut into 1/4-inch strips*
4 chicken legs with thighs (about
*   2 1/2 pounds), skinned and*
*   disjointed*
1/4 teaspoon salt
1/4 cup dry white wine or dry

*   vermouth*
1/2 cup Chicken Stock (page 19)
1/2 cup unsalted Italian tomato
*   purée*
1/2 teaspoon whole saffron, soaked
*   in 2 tablespoons boiling water*
2 tablespoons light cream
1 tablespoon cornstarch, dissolved
*   in 2 tablespoons water*
Minced parsley

1. Heat oil in well-seasoned iron skillet. Over medium-high heat, sauté garlic, onion, and green pepper until wilted, stirring often (about 2 minutes).
2. Rinse chicken and paper-dry. Prick all over with sharp-pronged fork. Sprinkle and rub with salt. Add to skillet in one layer over vegetables. Cook on both sides without browning until chicken loses its raw look (about 4 minutes).
3. Gather mixture in center of skillet. Pour wine around sides of skillet. Cook, without stirring, for 30 seconds. Combine stock with tomato purée; pour around sides of skillet. Cook, without stirring, for 30 seconds. Combine all ingredients. Stir in saffron-water mix. Turn chicken several times to coat. Bring to simmering point. Reduce heat. Cover and simmer for 35 minutes, turning and basting chicken with sauce twice at equal intervals.
4. Uncover. Turn up heat under skillet. Reduce sauce by one-third (about 5 minutes), turning and basting chicken every minute. Reduce heat. Pour in cream, stirring to blend. Drizzle in cornstarch mix, using just enough to lightly thicken sauce. Stir and simmer for 1 minute.
5. Transfer chicken pieces to warmed individual serving plates surrounded by colorful sauce. Sprinkle parsley over all, and serve at once.

Yield: **Serves 4**

CHICKEN WITH SUN-DRIED TOMATOES

When is a tomato *not* a tomato? When it's *sun-dried*. Until recently, this nature-dried delectable with a taste all its own has been a hard-to-find "designer" vegetable. To extend their unique-tasting shelf life, store them in your refrigerator in a tightly closed glass jar.

14 sun-dried tomatoes
About 1/3 cup boiling water
4 chicken legs with thighs (about 2 1/2 pounds), skinned and disjointed
2 tablespoons Italian olive oil
2 tablespoons Vegetable Mix (page 18)
1 tablespoon Savory Seasoning (page 15)
1 tablespoon each minced parsley

and fresh mint or dill
2 tablespoons cornstarch or arrowroot
2 tablespoons wine vinegar
1 cup coarsely chopped sweet green pepper
1/4 cup unsalted tomato juice
1/3 cup Chicken Stock (page 19)
1 tablespoon fresh lemon juice
1/4 teaspoon salt (optional)

1. Put tomatoes in colander; rinse under cold running water. Transfer to cup. Add enough boiling water to barely cover. Push tomatoes into water and let stand to soften (about 10 minutes). Drain, reserving liquid. Coarse-chop and set aside.
2. Rinse chicken and pat dry. Prick all over with sharp-pronged fork. Place in bowl. In cup, combine 1 tablespoon oil, Vegetable Mix, Savory Seasoning, and half the fresh herbs, blending well. Spread thick mixture over chicken. Cover and place in refrigerator for at least 2 hours. Sprinkle with cornstarch or arrowroot, turning to coat.
3. Heat remaining tablespoon of oil in a large well-seasoned iron skillet until hot. Over medium-high heat, sauté chicken until browned on each side. With spatula, scoop up and transfer to plate.
4. Remove skillet from heat. Pour in vinegar, scraping and loosening crusted bits. Cook until vinegar evaporates down to 1 teaspoon. Add green pepper, tomato juice, chopped tomatoes with cooking liquid, and stock. Bring to a boil. Return browned chicken to skillet, turning to coat. Bring to simmering point. Cover and simmer until tender (45 to 50 minutes), turning and spooning with sauce 3 times at equal intervals. Transfer chicken to warm serving plate. Cover to keep warm.
5. Add remaining tablespoon of fresh herbs. Turn up heat under skillet and cook and stir until sauce is thickened and reduced by 1/3. Stir in lemon juice. Taste for salt, adding it if desired. Dribble 3 tablespoons of sauce over chicken; spoon remainder around each serving.

Yield: **Serves 4**

CHICKEN CAKES

What crab meat is to crab cakes, chicken is to chicken cakes in this new way to prepare chicken breasts. Sprinkle with lemon juice and serve as a main course or hors d'oeuvre, or cover with its companion sauce for a more luxurious presentation.

For the cakes:

*1 pound skinned and boned
    chicken breasts, cut into strips
    1/4 inch wide and 1/2 inch
    long*
1 tablespoon dry sherry
*1 teaspoon flavorful honey, such as
    thyme*
1 tablespoon fresh lemon juice
*1 tablespoon Savory Seasoning
    (page 15)*
1/2 teaspoon aniseed, crushed
1/4 teaspoon salt

1 medium yam, peeled
*1 egg white, lightly beaten with 1
    tablespoon water*
2 tablespoons minced boiled ham
2 1/2 tablespoons cornstarch
*1 tablespoon minced fresh coriander
    or parsley*
2 tablespoons Italian olive oil
*2 tablespoons Vegetable Mix (page
    18), or 3 tablespoons minced
    shallot*
Parsley sprigs and lemon wedges

For the companion sauce:

1/4 cup reserved yams
3/4 cup Chicken Stock (page 19)
1/4 cup dry sherry
*1 tablespoon minced coriander or
    parsley*

*1 tablespoon frozen pineapple juice
    concentrate*
1/8 teaspoon salt
*2 teaspoons cornstarch dissolved in
    1 tablespoon water*

1. Place chicken in bowl. In cup, combine sherry, honey, and lemon juice and blend until honey thins down. Stir in seasonings. Pour over chicken, turning several times to coat. Refrigerate for 2 hours.
2. Cut yam into 1-inch chunks. Using food processor fitted with steel blade, fine-mince. Scrape into small heavy-bottomed saucepan. Add water to cover. Bring to boil. Reduce heat slightly and slow-boil for 10 minutes. Drain. Measure out 1 cup. Set aside.
3. Add egg mixture to chicken, blending well. Stir in 3/4 cup cooked yam (reserve balance for sauce), ham, cornstarch, and minced coriander or parsley.
4. Sauté in 2 batches or in 2 nonstick skillets. Heat 1 tablespoon oil in large skillet until hot. Strew 1 tablespoon Vegetable Mix across

skillet. For each cake, scoop up a heaping tablespoon of mixture and drop into skillet. Flatten with spatula to ⅜-inch thickness. Sauté over medium-high heat until crispy and brown on each side (about 6 minutes). Repeat procedure for balance of cakes. Keep warm in a preheated 250-degree oven as they're prepared.

5. Serve on a warm platter, garnished with parsley sprigs and lemon wedges, or prepare the following companion sauce.

1. In a small heavy-bottomed saucepan, combine reserved yam, stock, and sherry. Cook, uncovered, until reduced by one-third.

2. Stir in pineapple juice concentrate and salt. While stirring, dribble in cornstarch mixture, using just enough to thicken lightly. Simmer for 2 minutes.

3. Serve in gravyboat along with chicken cakes.

Yield: **8 to 10 cakes; about 1 cup sauce**

Variation: Serve as hors d'oeuvres. Allow 1 scant tablespoon mixture for each cake in Step 4. Cook until crispy. Sprinkle with lemon juice. Fold each cake over and secure with toothpicks. Serve hot sauce as a dip.

Yield: **for hors d'oeuvres 12 to 14 cakes**

CHICKEN CUTLETS WITH BUTTERNUT SQUASH

Minced butternut squash has the loveliest perfume and a gentle, sweet flavor that I've pointed up here with sweet spices, rosemary, a touch of sherry or champagne vinegar, and fruit juice. It is ambrosial spooned over these quickly sautéed tender chicken breasts.

1 to 1 1/4 pounds thin-sliced chicken breasts, skinned and boned
1/2 teaspoon each cinnamon, ground ginger, and freshly grated nutmeg
1 teaspoon dried rosemary, crushed
1/8 to 1/4 teaspoon salt
1/2 small butternut squash (about 3/4 pound), peeled and cut into 1/2-inch chunks
3 tablespoons minced shallot, or 2 tablespoons Vegetable Mix

(page 18)
2 tablespoons Italian olive oil
2 tablespoons sherry vinegar or champagne vinegar
2 tablespoons frozen orange juice concentrate
3/4 cup Chicken Stock (page 19)
1/2 teaspoon prepared Dijon mustard
1 tablespoon Light Choice sour cream or plain low-fat yogurt
Minced parsley or coriander

1. Wash and paper-dry chicken. In cup, combine spices, rosemary, and half the salt. Sprinkle and rub 1/2 of mixture over both sides of chicken. Set aside.
2. Fit food processor with steel blade. Add squash and shallot to workbowl and process until fine-minced. Measure out 1 1/2 tightly packed cups. Heat 1 tablespoon oil in heavy-bottomed saucepan. Add mixture and sauté for 2 minutes over moderate heat. Sprinkle with remaining spice mix. Add vinegar and cook for 1 minute. Combine orange juice concentrate and stock. Pour into saucepan, bring to a boil, and reduce heat to simmering. Cover and cook for 15 minutes, stirring once.
3. While sauce is simmering, heat remaining oil in large nonstick skillet. Over moderate heat, sauté chicken slices on both sides until lightly browned (about 7 minutes). Transfer to warm dish and cover to keep warm.
4. Pour cooked squash mix into blender and purée. Pour back into saucepan and stir in mustard and sour cream (or yogurt) over low

heat, taking care not to boil. Taste for salt, adding remaining ⅛ teaspoon if desired.

5. Serve chicken on individual warmed serving plates, spooned first with exuded juices from chicken, then napped with sauce. Spoon equal portions of sauce around chicken. Sprinkle with minced parsley or coriander.

Yield: **Serves 4**

OVEN-"FRIED" CHICKEN

This technique results in chicken just as crispy, tasty, and juicy as traditional fried chicken—even though it's never even been in the vicinity of a frying utensil. A how-did-you-ever-do-it? kind of dish, it's just right for those who must, or want, to break the fried-food habit. Or for those who just like good old-fashioned fried chicken. It *could* fool them!

2 tablespoons frozen orange juice concentrate
1 tablespoon unseasoned Oriental sesame oil
2 teaspoons low-sodium soy sauce
2 tablespoons dry sherry
2 teaspoons minced garlic
1/2 teaspoon mild curry powder
1 3-pound broiling chicken, skinned, wing tips removed, cut into eighths

1/3 to 1/2 cup Breading Mix (page 17)
1 tablespoon Italian olive oil
1 tablespoon sweet butter/margarine blend, cut into small pieces
2 tablespoons freshly grated Parmesan cheese
Juice of 1/2 lemon
Lemon wedges
Parsley sprigs

1. Prepare marinade by placing first six ingredients in large bowl, beating with fork to blend. With sharp-pronged fork, pierce chicken all over. Immerse in marinade and turn several times to coat. Cover and refrigerate for 2 hours or longer. Drain.
2. Sprinkle half Breading Mix onto large plate or sheet of wax paper. Lay chicken pieces over mixture, pressing to adhere. Sprinkle with remaining half-cup mix, coating evenly. Chill for 20 minutes to set.
3. Preheat oven to 450 degrees. Spread oil across non-aluminum metal baking pan large enough to hold chicken in one layer. Place pan in hot oven for 8 minutes. Quickly arrange drained pieces in hot pan without crowding. Reduce oven heat to 400 degrees. Bake chicken for 15 minutes.
4. Using spatula, scoop each chicken piece from pan and turn. Bake for 10 minutes. Dot with shortening and sprinkle with cheese. Bake for 15 minutes, piggybacking smaller pieces atop larger ones, if necessary, to prevent scorching. Turn and bake for 5 minutes longer. Sprinkle with lemon juice. Garnish with lemon wedges and parsley sprigs.

Yield: **Serves 4**

CHICKEN NUGGETS

For reasons I imagine scientists will discover one day, chicken close to the bone is more flavorful and succulent than chicken removed from the bone. So I bypass packaged chicken breasts, and opt to remove the breasts from two 3- to 3½-pound broiling chickens (a sharp knife and about 2 minutes does it). The result—chicken nuggets that outshine any of the commercial varieties. Serve as a main course or, pierced with cocktail picks, as an appetizer dipped in Barbecue Sauce (page 147). The remainder of the chicken goes into a second meal and my stock pot.

¼ cup dry sherry
1½ tablespoons frozen pineapple
    or orange juice concentrate
½ teaspoon dried cilantro
6 cloves, crushed
1¼ pounds chicken breasts,
    skinned and boned, cut into
    1-inch chunks
Scant ½ cup Breading Mix (page
    17)
1½ tablespoons Italian olive oil

3 tablespoons coarsely chopped
    shallot
2 teaspoons minced garlic
¼ pound snow-white fresh
    mushrooms, ends trimmed,
    damp-wiped, and sliced
⅓ cup Chicken Stock (page 19)
½ teaspoon sugar
¼ teaspoon salt
1 tablespoon minced parsley

1. In a bowl, combine and blend 2 tablespoons sherry, pineapple juice concentrate, cilantro, and cloves. Add chicken, turning several times to coat. Cover and refrigerate for 2 hours.
2. Sprinkle ⅓ of Breading Mix across a large sheet of wax paper. Drain chicken, reserving marinade. Lay chicken pieces over mixture, pressing to adhere. Sprinkle with remaining Mix, pressing into chicken all over. Transfer to plate and chill in freezer for 15 minutes.
3. Heat oil over medium-high heat in large nonstick skillet until hot. Add shallot and garlic. Sauté for 1 minute; then spread across skillet. Lay chicken atop mixture and cook, without stirring, for 2 minutes. Using spatula, turn chicken pieces. Add mushrooms. Sauté until chicken is browned all over, rolling when necessary.
4. Nestle chicken and mushrooms in center of skillet. Combine reserved marinade with stock. Add sugar, salt, parsley, and remaining 2 tablespoons sherry to mixture. Pour around sides of skillet. Turn up heat and bring to boil. Combine with chicken and cook until all liquid evaporates (about 2 minutes). Serve at once.

Yield: **Serves 4**

Note: For added zing, substitute 4 tablespoons Vegetable Mix and a dash of cayenne pepper (page 18) for shallot and garlic.

COUNTRY-KITCHEN CHICKEN WITH EGGPLANT SAUCE

Eggplant soaks up liquids like a sponge. Cooks don't like that, so they sprinkle it with salt and load it down with heavy weights to make it absorb less liquid. I don't. Instead I take advantage of the disadvantage, and let the vegetable absorb seasoned cooking liquids, which then naturally thicken into a mouth-watering sauce.

1 3-pound broiling chicken,
    skinned, wing tips removed,
    cut into eighths
1 tablespoon Savory Seasoning
    (page 15)
¼ cup each unbleached flour and
    fine-toasted bread crumbs,
    combined
2 teaspoons dried sage leaves,
    crushed, or 1 teaspoon rubbed
    sage
6 teaspoons Italian olive oil
2 tablespoons Vegetable Mix (page

18)
1 cup ½-inch cubes peeled
    eggplant
1 large onion, coarsely chopped
⅓ cup dry red wine
1 cup unsalted Italian tomatoes,
    chopped
8 sprigs parsley tied together with
    white cotton thread
¼ teaspoon salt
3 tablespoons freshly grated
    Parmesan cheese

1. Preheat oven to 350 degrees. Rinse chicken and dry completely with paper toweling. Sprinkle and rub all over with Savory Seasoning. In a cup, combine flour with bread crumbs and sage.
2. Tear off a large sheet of wax paper. Sprinkle ⅓ flour mix across sheet. Lay chicken pieces over mixture, pressing to adhere. Sprinkle ⅓ mix over chicken, pressing and turning several times to coat evenly, using remaining mix if necessary.
3. Heat 2 teaspoons oil in a well-seasoned iron skillet over medium-high heat. Lightly brown chicken, half at a time, on both sides. Transfer to a plate. Heat 2 teaspoons oil in skillet. Repeat procedure, transferring second batch to plate.
4. Add remaining 2 teaspoons oil to skillet. Sauté Vegetable Mix, eggplant, and onion until lightly browned, taking care not to scorch. Add wine. Cook for 1 minute. Pour in tomatoes and drop in parsley bundle. Bring to a boil.

5. Return chicken to skillet, turning to coat. Cover, bring to a boil; then reduce heat to simmering. Cook on top of stove for 2 minutes. Place in center section of preheated oven and bake for 20 minutes. Sprinkle with salt. Turn chicken and baste. Re-cover and bake until tender (25 to 30 minutes).

6. Uncover. Discard parsley after pressing out juices. Spoon thick sauce over chicken. Sprinkle with Parmesan cheese. Re-cover and let stand for 5 minutes. Serve hot.

Yield: **Serves 4**

ORANGE-SAUCED CHICKEN

Here is an exceptional marinade that grows into a sauce. The essences of orange and sherry build to full stature with onion, stock, and parsley. Milk and a hint of cream thicken it into a lovely new-tasting orange sauce.

For the marinade:

2 tablespoons frozen orange juice
    concentrate
2 tablespoons dry sherry
½ teaspoon mild curry powder

1 teaspoon dried tarragon leaves,
    crumbled
3 whole cloves, crushed

For the chicken and sauce:

1 pound chicken breasts,
    thin-sliced, boned, and
    skinned
½ cup coarsely chopped onion
½ cup Chicken Stock (page 19)
¼ teaspoon salt
1 tablespoon minced parsley
½ cup milk
2 tablespoons light cream

1 tablespoon each sweet
    butter/margarine blend and
    Italian olive oil
4 large cloves garlic, peeled and
    halved
2 teaspoons cornstarch, dissolved in
    1 tablespoon water
Freshly ground black or white
    pepper

1. In medium bowl, combine concentrate, sherry, curry powder, ½ teaspoon tarragon, and cloves. Beat with fork to blend. Add chicken, turning several times to coat. Marinate at room temperature for 30 minutes, or cover and refrigerate for several hours.

2. Drain each slice of chicken, reserving marinade. Then lay on doubled sheet of paper toweling. Blot lightly with another sheet of paper. Set aside.

3. Pour reserved marinade into small heavy-bottomed saucepan. Add onion, stock, salt, remaining ½ teaspoon tarragon, and parsley. Bring to a boil. Reduce heat to simmering. Cook, uncovered, for 5 minutes. Add milk and cream. Stir and simmer for 2 minutes. Remove from heat.

4. Heat shortening and oil over medium heat in large nonstick skillet. When hot, add garlic halves. Stir garlic around skillet, cooking for

1½ minutes; discard. Arrange chicken in one layer in skillet. Raise heat slightly and sauté on each side for 2 minutes. Pour in hot sauce, turning chicken several times to coat. Lower heat and simmer for 21 minutes more.

5. Dribble in 1 teaspoon cornstarch mix, stirring sauce continually. (Dribble in only enough of remaining mixture to make a lightly thickened sauce.) Simmer for 1 minute. Sprinkle with pepper.

6. Serve chicken slices on warmed individual plates. Spoon equal amounts of sauce around each serving.

Yield: **Serves 4**

Serving suggestion: Just-steamed broccoli florets, lightly seasoned with a sweet butter/margarine blend and freshly grated nutmeg, make a delightful accompaniment.

HOLIDAY CORNISH HENS

How do you prepare a savory holiday-style stuffing without using fat-laden sausage and pounds of butter? You start with an exceptional corn bread, accent it with fruity dried apricots, and complement it with herbs, spices, stock, and fruit juice. If you keep corn bread in your freezer, as I do, you can enjoy this holiday stuffing any day, with either chicken or turkey as well.

For the stuffing:

12 dried unsulphured apricot
 halves
6 cups Dinner Corn bread (page
 166), cut in 1/2-inch cubes
 and toasted
2 tablespoons each Italian olive oil
 and sweet butter/margarine
 blend
1/2 cup each minced celery and
 onion
1/2 teaspoon each dried thyme and
 cinnamon

1 1/2 teaspoons dried sage, crushed
1/4 cup minced boiled ham
 (optional)
1/3 cup coarsely chopped roasted
 chestnuts, or canned, drained,
 imported unseasoned chestnuts
2 tablespoons minced parsley
about 1 cup Chicken Stock (page
 19), warmed
1/3 cup unsweetened apple juice
1 egg, well beaten with fork

For the hens and gravy:

4 1-pound Cornish hens
1 teaspoon each dried thyme and
 crushed sage leaves, combined
3 tablespoons minced shallot
1 tablespoon minced garlic
1 tablespoon sweet
 butter/margarine blend, cut

 into small pieces
1 tablespoon Italian olive oil
1/2 cup each Chicken Stock (page
 19) and dry sherry, combined
1 recipe Cranberry Gravy (page
 151)
Crisp watercress sprigs

1. To prepare stuffing, rinse apricots and place in small cup. Add just enough boiling water to cover. Let soak for 30 minutes. Squeeze out and cut into small pieces. Set aside.
2. Place corn bread in large bowl. Heat oil mixture in small nonstick skillet until hot. Over moderate heat, sauté celery and onion until wilted without browning. Sprinkle in thyme, cinnamon, and sage; sauté for 30 seconds. Add ham and chestnuts. Sauté for 1 minute more. Gently fold mix into corn bread; stir in drained apricots and parsley.

3. Combine ½ cup stock with apple juice and beaten egg. While stirring, pour slowly into stuffing. Let stand for 10 minutes to absorb. Add enough of remaining stock mix to make a mixture that is moist but not sticky.

4. Preheat oven to 400 degrees.

5. To prepare hens, rinse inside and out and dry thoroughly with paper toweling. Rub ¼ teaspoon combined herbs into each hen cavity. Fill with stuffing, pressing gently without overpacking. Combine shallot and garlic. Carefully lift up skin on each side of cavity on both hens and push mixture in, allowing 1 tablespoon for each hen. Flatten down so that most of the breast area is filled evenly. Close cavities with small skewers and white cotton thread. Truss each bird so that wings and legs hug body. Place remaining stuffing in lightly greased 8-inch loaf pan. Dot with 1 teaspoon sweet butter/margarine blend and cover tightly with aluminum foil. Set stuffing aside.

6. Place hens on rack in roasting pan, breasts up. Brush with oil; sprinkle and rub with remaining teaspoon herbs. Cover tightly with heavy-duty aluminum foil. Roast in center section of oven for 20 minutes. Reduce heat to 350 degrees. Baste with ¼ cup stock and sherry mixture. Re-cover and roast for 30 minutes more. Repeat basting procedure once more.

7. Put loaf pan of stuffing in oven. Repeat basting procedure for hens every 15 minutes twice more, for a total of 80 minutes roasting time. Baste again and roast, uncovered, for 10 minutes. Remove birds and loaf pan from oven. Pour pan juices from hens into a cup and set aside.

8. While hens continue to roast, prepare Cranberry Gravy, adding reserved pan juices from hens before milk is incorporated in last step of recipe.

9. To serve, arrange watercress around sides of warmed platter. Remove skewers and trussing from hens. Place birds in center of platter. Drizzle with 2 tablespoons gravy. Pour remaining gravy in gravyboat and serve along with hens and extra stuffing.

Yield: **Hens serve 4, with extra stuffing**

Notes:

1. If ham is not used in stuffing, you may want to add ¼ teaspoon salt in Step 2.

2. Uncooked stuffing is enough to fill an 8- to 10-pound turkey.

Serving suggestions: Try Cornish hens with my Potato and Apple Medley (page 52), or with Brussels sprouts, peas, or broccoli, seasoned with a touch of sweet butter/margarine blend, freshly grated nutmeg, minced parsley or mint, and a light sprinkling of salt.

LEMON CHICKEN WITH PORCINI MUSHROOMS

To the growing list of cross-cultural dishes add this tender poached chicken bathed in a tart Chinese lemon sauce that reaches a new height of sophistication with Italian porcini mushrooms.

For the chicken:

2 whole chicken breasts with bone (about 1 1/4 pounds), skinned
1 rib celery, thinly sliced
1 small carrot, peeled and thinly sliced
1 small onion, peeled and sliced
1 fresh thyme sprig, or 1/4 teaspoon dried thyme
3 cups water
1 bay leaf
8 sprigs parsley

For the sauce:

1/2 ounce dried porcini mushrooms
1 tablespoon peanut oil
2 tablespoons well-scrubbed fresh ginger, cut into 1/8-inch strips
1 small sweet red pepper, seeded, cut into 1/4-inch strips
4 scallions, including 1 inch of green part, trimmed, thinly sliced on the diagonal
1 tablespoon lemon rind, cut into 1/8-inch strips
1/3 cup fresh lemon juice
3/4 cup poaching liquid
2 teaspoons sugar
1/4 teaspoon salt
1 teaspoon rice wine vinegar
2 teaspoons cornstarch, dissolved in 1 tablespoon poaching liquid
1/2 teaspoon lemon extract (optional)
Lemon slices

1. Place chicken in wide heavy-bottomed saucepan or kettle. Add balance of ingredients, pushing parsley and bay leaf into liquid. Bring to a boil. Reduce heat to simmering. Cover and simmer until chicken is tender (40 to 45 minutes). Uncover partially, letting chicken cool in liquid. Using slotted spoon, transfer chicken to cutting board. Cover loosely with wax paper.
2. Pour remaining contents of saucepan through fine sieve or chinois with bowl underneath, pressing out juices. Skim off any fat (it will be negligible). Measure out 1 cup, reserving balance. When chicken has cooled down, cut into 1-inch pieces with sharp knife. Set aside.

3. Rinse mushrooms. Place in a cup. Add enough boiling water to barely cover. Let soak for 30 minutes. Squeeze out and chop coarsely.
4. Heat oil in a wok or nonstick skillet until hot (a wok is preferable because it cooks ingredients rapidly and permits chicken pieces to spread out with minimal breakage). Add ginger and sauté for 15 seconds. Add red pepper, scallions, and squeezed-out mushrooms. Sprinkle in lemon rind.
5. Combine lemon juice, ¾ cup poaching liquid, sugar, salt, and vinegar. Pour around sides of wok or skillet. Gently combine chicken with mixture, stirring with a large spoon. Bring to a boil. Dribble cornstarch mix around sides of wok or skillet. Gently combine chicken with mixture, stirring with large spoon. Cook over medium-high heat only until heated through. Taste for lemon seasoning. If you prefer a stronger lemon flavor, sprinkle in lemon extract, combining carefully. Serve on individual warmed plates garnished with lemon slices.

Yield: **Serves 4**

BRAISED CHICKEN WITH PLUMS

Purple plums are traditionally associated with tortes and pies and an abundance of sugar. Here, combined with chicken, cranberries, and apples, they work as a natural gravy thickener that adds subtle flavor to a spice-infused sauce. I blanche summer purple plums for 30 seconds in boiling water, then freeze them for use year-round.

1 large Granny Smith apple, peeled, cored, and coarsely chopped
1/2 cup fresh cranberries, rinsed
3/4 pound small purple plums, peeled, pitted, and cut into small pieces
2 tablespoons frozen orange juice concentrate
5 sprigs parsley, tied into a neat bundle with white cotton thread
1/8 teaspoon allspice
1 tablespoon flavorful honey, such as thyme

1 cup water
1 3 1/2-pound broiling chicken, skinned, cut into eighths
1/2 teaspoon cinnamon
1 teaspoon ground ginger
1/4 teaspoon salt
1 teaspoon dried rosemary, finely crushed
1 1/2 tablespoons Italian olive oil
3 tablespoons minced shallot
1 cup Chicken Stock (page 19) or water
1 to 2 tablespoons fresh lemon juice
Orange slices and minced parsley

1. Combine first eight ingredients in heavy-bottomed 1¾-quart saucepan. Bring to a boil. Cover partially and cook over low heat for 30 minutes. Uncover and cook over moderate heat until very thick (about 30 minutes). Discard parsley bundle; set aside. (Mixture may be prepared a day ahead and refrigerated.)
2. Rinse and paper-dry chicken. Prick all over with a sharp-pronged fork. In a cup, combine and blend spices, salt, and rosemary. Sprinkle and rub on chicken.
3. Heat a large well-seasoned iron skillet with oil until hot. Strew shallots across skillet. Sauté for 1 minute over medium-high heat. Arrange chicken in one layer over shallots. Cook for 3 minutes on each side, taking care not to scorch. Pour stock or water around sides of skillet and bring to a boil. Reduce heat to simmering, cover, and braise until tender (45 to 50 minutes), turning and basting with juices 3 times at equal intervals. Transfer chicken to a warm serving plate; cover to keep warm.

4. Skim any fat from pan juices. Over medium-high heat, reduce juices by half. Add fruit mixture and 1 tablespoon lemon juice. Bring to simmering point. Simmer, uncovered, over moderate heat for 5 minutes. Taste and add remaining lemon juice if desired.

5. Spoon half the sauce onto warmed serving platter. Arrange chicken over sauce. Ladle remaining sauce over chicken. Garnish with orange slices and minced parsley.

Yield: **Serves 4**

Serving suggestion: This chicken goes well with my Eight-Minute Kasha (page 60) or Wild Rice and Barley Medley (page 63).

BATTER-BAKED CHICKEN WITH VEGETABLE MÉLANGE

The batter-cloaked chicken is oven-baked, the vegetables are quick-sautéed, and the combination is an eye-catching array of colors.

For the chicken:

2 tablespoons peanut oil
1 small egg yolk
1/3 cup each Chicken Stock (page 19) and water
1 teaspoon Worcestershire sauce
1 tablespoon frozen apple juice concentrate
1/2 teaspoon each ground ginger and mild curry powder

1/8 teaspoon salt
About 1/2 cup unbleached flour
1 1/2 teaspoons non-aluminum baking powder
1 3- to 3 1/2-pound broiling chicken, skinned, wing tips removed, cut into eighths
1/2 lemon, plus lemon wedges for garnish

For the vegetables:

1 tablespoon Italian olive oil
2 teaspoons minced fresh ginger
3 medium zucchini, scrubbed, cut into 1/2-inch cubes
1 medium onion, thin-sliced, separated into rings
1 small sweet red pepper, seeded, cut into 1/4-inch strips

1/4 pound snow-white fresh mushrooms, ends trimmed, damp-wiped, sliced
1 1/2 teaspoons mild curry powder
1/8 teaspoon salt
1 tablespoon minced fresh coriander
Black pepper to taste

1. Preheat oven to 450 degrees. Spread oil across non-aluminum metal baking pan large enough to hold chicken in one layer. Place pan in lower section of hot oven for 7 minutes.
2. In a small bowl, whisk together egg yolk, stock, water, Worcesershire sauce, concentrate, and seasonings. In another bowl, place flour and baking powder. Slowly whisk stock mixture into dry ingredients. Mixture should be thick.
3. Wash chicken and dry thoroughly with paper toweling. Prick all over with sharp-pronged fork. Immerse in batter for 5 minutes. Lift

out and drain. Take hot pan out of oven. Arrange chicken across pan without crowding. Bake for 15 minutes. Reduce heat to 400 degrees. Bake for 15 minutes more. Using metal spatula, scoop up each piece and turn. Return to oven for 10 minutes. Turn again carefully. Return to oven until crispy and well browned (5 to 10 minutes).

4. After chicken has baked for 30 minutes, sauté vegetables. In 2 large nonstick skillets, heat oil until quite hot. Add ginger and sauté for 1 minute over moderately high heat. Add zucchini, onion, and red pepper; sauté for 5 minutes, stirring every 30 seconds. Add mushrooms. Sprinkle with seasonings, stir, and continue sautéing until zucchini is still crisp but tender (about 3 minutes). Remove from heat and leave uncovered.

5. Scoop up crisp chicken and cracklings from pan. Arrange in a circle on outer edges of warm serving plate. Reheat vegetables briefly. Spoon onto center of circle. Sprinkle chicken with juice from ½ lemon, and sprinkle vegetables with coriander and pepper. Garnish with lemon wedges.

Yield: **Serves 4**

Serving suggestion: Fresh Horseradish Sauce (page 152) adds a nice tang to this dish.

CLAY-POT CHICKEN

What I like best about clay-pot cooking is its infallible explosive heartiness—the burst of rich flavors from the food itself, the aromatic magnificence of its seasonings.

1 recipe Juniper Berry Marinade
  (page 154)
1 3½-pound broiling chicken,
  skinned
2 teaspoons each sweet
  butter/margarine blend and
  Italian olive oil, combined
1 large onion, thinly sliced
4 snow-white fresh mushrooms,

ends trimmed, damp-wiped,
  thinly sliced
10 large cloves garlic, peeled and
  cut into thirds
1 cup peeled and ½-inch diced
  yellow wax turnip
About 8 large dill sprigs
Chopped fresh dill

1. Soak clay pot (including cover) in tepid water for 20 to 30 minutes.
2. Prepare marinade in a wide bowl. Cut chicken down spine and spread out butterfly-fashion. Prick all over with sharp-pronged fork. Immerse in marinade, turning several times to coat inside and out. Cover and marinate in refrigerator for 4 to 5 hours, returning it to room temperature before cooking.
3. Put half the shortening mix into a nonstick skillet. Over moderate heat, sauté onion and mushrooms for 3 minutes, stirring continually. Empty clay pot; do not dry. Spoon half sautéed mixture across ridged bottom section. Transfer balance to a small plate. Sauté garlic and turnip in remaining shortening mix for 2 minutes. Spread half onto onion mixture.
4. Drain chicken, reserving marinade. Open out fully and lay over vegetables, bony side down. Strew remaining onion and turnip mix over chicken. Then pour marinade evenly over everything. Arrange as many dill sprigs as necessary to cover all.
5. Position rack in bottom third of oven. Set thermostat at 400 degrees. Place pot on rack and bake for 1 hour and 20 minutes. Uncover, moving your head to the side as the steam momentarily surges upward. Finished chicken will be lightly browned, juicy, and exceptionally tender.
6. Using two large spoons, gently press sections of bird apart into serving pieces and arrange on warmed individual serving dishes. Sprinkle with chopped dill and serve.

Yield: **Serves 4**

Serving suggestion: Try this with my Carrot/Cauliflower Purée (page 156).

CHICKEN IN CREAMY SPICE SAUCE

Have you ever wondered why the sauces in the great restaurants are as smooth as silk? It's because they're whisked or stirred from start to finish. This simple cooking technique will produce four-star-restaurant results every time.

1 tablespoon each Italian olive oil and sweet butter/margarine blend

1 teaspoon each mild curry powder and ground coriander

Pinch cayenne pepper

1 tablespoon Vegetable Mix (page 18)

3 tablespoons trimmed, damp-wiped, and coarsely chopped snow-white fresh mushrooms

3 tablespoons unbleached flour

2 tablespoons dry sherry

1 ripe medium tomato, seeded,

skinned, and coarsely chopped

about 1¼ cups Chicken Stock (page 19)

2 cups 1-inch cubed tender and moist cooked chicken

2 tablespoons unsalted chopped pimentos, drained

¼ teaspoon salt

2 tablespoons Light Choice sour cream or plain low-fat yogurt

¼ cup loosely packed and coarsely chopped fresh basil, or 2 tablespoons chopped just-snipped fresh dill

1. In heavy-bottomed 2-quart saucepan, combine oil and shortening over moderate heat. Heat until it foams. Sprinkle in spices. Cook for 30 seconds. Add Vegetable Mix and mushrooms. Sauté until mushrooms begin to wilt.

2. Stir in flour. Using rapid strokes, stir and cook for 1 minute (mixture will be thick). Combine with sherry; cook for 30 seconds. Stir in tomato. Then gradually blend in stock, using enough to make a fairly thick sauce.

3. Fold in chicken and pimentos. Add salt. Partially cover and simmer over low heat for 2 minutes. Remove from stove and fold in sour cream or yogurt and fresh herbs. Serve immediately on warmed individual plates over a bed of just-cooked rice.

Yield: **Serves 4**

CHICKEN FETTUCINI

The bright taste of the fragrant, smooth-textured sauce for this chicken and pasta dish is totally reliant on the freshness of the ingredients. The entire recipe is quick to make, so it tastes best when prepared just before serving time.

½ pound snow-white fresh mushrooms, damp-wiped, quartered, and thinly sliced

1 medium zucchini, well scrubbed, cut into ½-inch cubes

1 large sweet red pepper, seeded, cut into 2-inch strips

¾ pound skinned and boned chicken breasts, cut into ¼-inch pieces

¼ teaspoon each salt and freshly grated nutmeg

½ teaspoon mild curry powder

1½ tablespoons Italian olive oil

1 tablespoon Vegetable Mix (page 18)

⅔ cup Chicken Stock (page 19)

½ cup unsalted Italian tomato purée

1½ teaspoons prepared Dijon mustard, preferably without salt

1 tablespoon fresh lemon juice

¼ cup milk

2 tablespoons whipping cream or Light Choice sour cream

¾ cup loosely packed coarsely chopped, rinsed, fresh basil leaves

⅓ cup freshly grated Parmesan cheese

6 ounces fettucini

2 teaspoons arrowroot or cornstarch

Freshly ground white or black pepper

1. Place mushrooms, zucchini, and pepper in large heavy-bottomed saucepan. Add water to cover (about 2 cups) and bring to a boil. Boil briskly, uncovered, for 2 minutes, pushing vegetables into liquid several times. Drain through strainer, reserving liquid. Set solids and liquid aside.

2. Rinse chicken under cold running water. Dry thoroughly with paper toweling. In a cup, combine seasonings; sprinkle and rub all over chicken. Cut into ½-inch pieces.

3. Heat oil in well-seasoned iron skillet. Over moderate heat, sauté Vegetable Mix for 1 minute. Spread across skillet. Arrange chicken pieces in one layer over it. Sauté over medium-high heat, stirring often, until lightly browned (about 5 minutes). Pour stock around sides of skillet. Combine with chicken and cook for 1 minute.

4. In a cup, combine tomato purée with mustard and lemon juice.

Add to skillet. Bring to simmering point. Add cream (or sour cream) and ½ cup basil. Stir to blend. Then combine with cooked vegetables and ¼ cup cheese. Simmer for 5 minutes.

5. While sauce is being prepared, cook fettucini. Place reserved vegetable liquid in large pot; add 2 cups water. Bring to boil. Add fettucini, stirring to separate. Cook for 8 minutes. (If using fresh fettucini, cook for 3 to 4 minutes.)

6. To thicken sauce, combine arrowroot (or cornstarch) in a cup with remaining stock, stirring until very smooth. Drizzle into sauce, stirring until lightly thickened.

7. Drain pasta and transfer to warmed serving bowl. Spoon in sauce, tossing to coat. Sprinkle with remaining cheese and basil. Top with freshly ground pepper.

Yield: **Serves 4**

Serving suggestions: This pasta goes well with Savoy Salad (page 176) or Bok Choy Salad (page 179).

CHICKEN PAELLA WITH ARTICHOKES AND MUSHROOMS

The chicken and rice are partially cooked in stock, tomatoes, and seasonings, then assembled with artichokes to make an exciting American-style paella.

1/2 ounce imported dried mushrooms (dark variety); see Note

1 9-ounce box frozen artichoke hearts

2 small (1-pound) boned and skinned chicken breasts, halved and flattened

4 teaspoons Savory Seasoning (page 15)

4 teaspoons Italian olive oil

2 tablespoons fresh lemon juice

3 tablespoons Vegetable Mix (page 18)

1/2 coarsely chopped sweet green

pepper

3/4 cup long-grain rice

1 1/4 cups Chicken Stock (page 19)

1 cup imported unsalted Italian plum tomatoes, drained and coarsely chopped

1 teaspoon prepared Dijon mustard, preferably without salt

1/4 teaspoon salt

Dash cayenne pepper

2 tablespoons minced parsley

3 tablespoons freshly grated Parmesan cheese

1. Rinse mushrooms, break up, and place in cup. Add enough boiling water to barely cover and soak until softened. Squeeze out, reserving 2 tablespoons soaking liquid. Set aside.

2. Place artichokes in small heavy-bottomed saucepan. Add 1/4 cup water. Bring to a boil. Reduce heat to simmering and cook for 6 minutes, breaking up hearts after 3 minutes. Drain. Cut away tough sections; coarse-chop tender portions.

3. Rinse chicken and paper-dry. Cut into 1-inch pieces. Sprinkle all over with 2 teaspoons Savory Seasoning. Heat 2 teaspoons oil in large nonstick skillet. Over medium-high heat, sauté until lightly browned all over (about 4 minutes). Transfer to a plate. Sprinkle with lemon juice, turning to coat.

4. Heat remaining 2 teaspoons oil in skillet. Over medium heat, sauté Vegetable Mix and green pepper until limp. Stir in remaining 2 teaspoons Savory Seasoning. Combine rice with mixture, stirring to coat. Cook for 1 minute. Add 1 cup stock, tomatoes, mustard, mushrooms, and reserved soaking liquid. Bring to a boil, then reduce heat to simmering. Cover tightly and cook until all liquid is absorbed and rice is almost tender, stirring twice at equal intervals. Fold in artichokes; sprinkle with salt and cayenne and combine with parsley.

5. Preheat oven to 350 degrees. Lightly oil a 2-quart decorative ovenproof casserole. Spread with half the rice mixture. Arrange chicken breasts side by side in one layer. Pour in exuded juices from chicken. Sprinkle with half the Parmesan cheese. Cover with balance of rice mix. Sprinkle with remaining cheese. Then cover and bake in center section of oven for 20 minutes. Uncover, pour remaining ¼ cup stock over all, and return to oven for 15 minutes.

6. Serve the paella directly from casserole at the table.

Yield: **Serves 4 to 5**

Note: These mushrooms are labeled "Imported Dried Mushrooms" and are available in supermarkets. They are packed in ½-ounce clear plastic boxes for easy identification of the light or dark variety.

CHICKEN WITH NEW MOUSSELINE SAUCE

Chicken juices and solids are whirred in your blender just before serving to produce an intriguing sauce that suggests the smoothness of a mousseline. But there's no whipped cream or eggs, making a dish that's very low in calories but very high in satisfaction.

4 chicken legs with thighs (about 2½ pounds), skinned and disjointed
1½ tablespoons Savory Seasoning (page 15)
4 teaspoons Italian olive oil
1 medium onion, coarsely chopped
2 teaspoons minced garlic
1 teaspoon finely minced fresh ginger

2 teaspoons white wine Worcestershire sauce
⅓ cup fresh cranberries
⅓ cup unsweetened apple juice
¼ teaspoon salt
Florets from 8 sprigs parsley
1 cup shelled fresh peas
2 teaspoons sweet butter/margarine blend
1 cup just-cooked rice or couscous

1. Rinse chicken and paper-dry. With a sharp-pronged fork, pierce skin all over. Sprinkle and rub with Savory Seasoning.
2. Heat oil in well-seasoned iron skillet until hot. Strew onion, garlic, and ginger across skillet. Sauté over moderate heat for 2 minutes. Arrange chicken over mixture. Raise heat and lightly brown on each side for 3 minutes.
3. Pour Worcestershire sauce around sides of skillet. Cook for 30 seconds. Add cranberries, apple juice, half the salt, and parsley. Bring to a boil. Turn chicken pieces several times to coat. Reduce heat to simmering. Cover and cook for 50 minutes, basting with sauce and turning four times at equal intervals. When cooking time is completed, baste with sauce, re-cover, and let rest for 10 minutes.
4. Steam peas or cook in rapidly boiling water. Drain. Transfer to a small saucepan, stir in shortening, and cover.
5. Reheat chicken briefly. Transfer with slotted spoon to center of warm serving platter. Tent with foil to keep warm. Pour sauce into food blender. Add remaining ⅛ teaspoon salt and purée on high speed until frothy.
6. Spoon rice or couscous around chicken. Arrange peas over it. Pour sauce over chicken and serve at once.

Yield: **Serves 4**

POACHED CHICKEN IN GREEN SAUCE

Tender chicken breasts are brought together with fresh sweet basil and bitter-edged endive, then poached until tender. The sauce is puréed and faintly seasoned with spices for a final gourmet touch.

2 whole chicken breasts with bone, skinned

2 small ribs celery, thin-sliced

2 medium Belgian endives, trimmed and thin-sliced

1 cup rinsed, coarsely chopped, and firmly packed fresh basil leaves

1/4 teaspoon dried thyme

1/2 cup dry white wine or vermouth

1 cup water or Chicken Stock (page 19)

6 whole peppercorns

1/4 teaspoon each mild curry powder and freshly grated nutmeg

1/4 teaspoon salt

3 tablespoons Light Choice sour cream or plain low-fat yogurt

Pinch sugar (optional)

1 tablespoon sweet butter/margarine blend

1/4 pound snow-white fresh mushrooms, damp-wiped, thin-sliced

2 tablespoons minced sweet red pepper or unsalted drained pimentos for garnish

1. Place chicken, meaty side down, in large heavy-bottomed saucepan. Add celery, endives, basil, thyme, wine, stock, and peppercorns. Bring to a boil. Cook for 2 minutes, skimming foam that rinses to the top. Reduce heat to simmering. Cover and cook for 40 minutes, pushing vegetables into liquid and stirring from time to time. Let stand, partially covered, for 20 minutes so chicken absorbs flavors. Transfer chicken to carving board. With sharp serrated knife, cut into 1-inch chunks. Tent with aluminum foil to keep warm.

2. Place saucepan over high heat and reduce liquid to 1 cup. Let cool for 5 minutes. Pour contents of saucepan into food blender and purée on high speed. Return to saucepan. Whisk in spices and salt. Simmer for 2 minutes. Then whisk in sour cream or yogurt. Heat to just under simmering point. Taste. Add the pinch of sugar if yogurt is used. Gently stir in chicken and remove from heat.

3. Heat shortening in small nonstick skillet until hot. Add mushrooms and sauté over medium-high heat, stirring often, for 3 minutes. Add to chicken and stir gently. Reheat briefly, taking care not to boil.

4. Ladle into warm serving bowls and top with minced pepper or pimentos.

Yield: **Serves 4**

ORIENTAL CHICKEN SAUTÉ

What especially intrigues many food lovers about Oriental cuisine is its combination of textures within a single dish. Here the crispness of fresh bok choy counterpoints the softness of apricots. Oriental parsley (fresh coriander) gives the dish an authentic garnish.

For the marinade:

1 tablespoon unseasoned Oriental
  sesame oil
1 tablespoon Savory Seasoning
  (page 15)
2 1/2 tablespoons fresh lime or

lemon juice
1 1/2 tablespoons frozen pineapple
  juice concentrate
1 tablespoon cornstarch
1 1/2 tablespoons water

For the chicken:

2 small boned and skinned chicken
  breasts (total weight about
  1 1/4 pounds), cut into
  1/2-inch pieces
12 dried unsulphured apricot
  halves
2 tablespoons peanut or olive oil
2 teaspoons each minced garlic and

fresh ginger
1 cup 1/2-inch strips fresh bok choy
1 medium sweet red pepper, seeded,
  cut into 1/4-inch strips
1/3 cup Chicken Stock (page 19)
1/4 cup dry sherry
2 tablespoons chopped fresh
  coriander

1. In a large bowl, combine all marinade ingredients, beating with fork to blend. Rinse and dry chicken. Add to marinade, turning several times to coat. Cover and let stand at room temperature for 1 hour, or refrigerate for several hours.
2. Rinse apricots. Place in a cup and add enough boiling water to cover. Let stand for 30 minutes. Squeeze out water and chop.
3. Heat half the oil in wok or large well-seasoned iron skillet. Add half the garlic and half the ginger, and stir-fry for 30 seconds. Drain chicken and quickly combine with mixture. Then spread across pan and cook over high heat for 30 seconds without stirring. Continue to sauté, arranging chicken pieces across pan each time they're stirred, until all pieces are lightly browned (about 5 minutes). Transfer to plate.
4. Heat remaining oil in pan; add remaining garlic and ginger, and

stir-fry for 30 seconds. Combine bok choy and pepper with mixture, and stir-fry until slightly softened but still crunchy (about 4 minutes).

5. Return chicken to pan; add apricots and mix well. Pour stock around sides of pan and stir-fry for 1 minute. Sauce should be bubbling and lightly thickened. Drizzle sherry around sides of pan and stir-fry for 30 seconds longer.

6. Serve chicken immediately on warmed plates, sprinkled with chopped coriander.

Yield: **Serves 4**

BAKED CHICKEN WITH PIQUANT SAUCE

Once you've been surprised by this crispy chicken—it tastes *fried!*—with its creamy sauce, you'll probably exclaim, "What did I ever see in breaded fried chicken with heavy fat-laden gravy!" That's why I created this recipe.

For the chicken:

2 tablespoons frozen apple juice concentrate

1 tablespoon Worcestershire sauce

3 tablespoons Chicken Stock (page 19)

3 tablespoons dry sherry

2 tablespoons minced shallot

1 teaspoon unsalted prepared Dijon mustard

2 teaspoons dried rosemary, crushed

1 3-pound broiling chicken, skinned, wing tips removed, cut into eighths

1/3 to 1/2 cup Breading Mix (page 17)

2 tablespoons Italian olive oil

1 tablespoon sweet butter/margarine blend, cut into small pieces

2 tablespoons freshly grated sharp cheddar cheese

Orange slices

Watercress sprigs

For the sauce:

Reserved marinade

2 tablespoons frozen apple juice concentrate

1/3 to 1/2 cup Chicken Stock (page 19)

1 tablespoon Worcestershire sauce

2 tablespoons minced fresh coriander

2 tablespoons dry sherry

1/8 to 1/4 teaspoon salt

1 1/2 tablespoons cornstarch dissolved in 1 1/2 tablespoons Chicken Stock or water

1. Prepare marinade by placing first 7 ingredients in large bowl, beating with fork to blend. With sharp-pronged fork, pierce chicken all over. Immerse in marinade, and turn several times to coat. Cover and refrigerate for 2 hours or longer. Drain, reserving marinade.

2. Sprinkle half Breading Mix onto large plate or sheet of wax paper. Arrange chicken pieces over mixture, pressing to adhere. Sprinkle with remaining half-cup mix, coating evenly. Chill for 20 minutes to set.

3. Preheat oven to 450 degrees. Spread oil across non-aluminum metal baking pan large enough to hold chicken in one layer. Place pan in hot oven for 7 minutes. Quickly arrange coated chicken in pan without crowding. Reduce oven heat to 400 degrees. Bake chicken for 15 minutes.

4. Using spatula, scoop up each chicken piece from pan and turn. Bake for 10 minutes. Dot each piece with shortening and sprinkle with cheese. Bake for 15 minutes, piggybacking smaller pieces over larger ones, if necessary, to prevent scorching. Turn and bake for 5 minutes longer.

5. While chicken bakes, prepare sauce. Pour reserved marinade into small heavy-bottomed saucepan. Bring to simmering point. Cook, uncovered, for 5 minutes. Strain into a cup, pressing out juices. Return to rinsed-out saucepan. Add remaining ingredients, except cornstarch mixture. There should be 1 cup; if less, add more stock. (Sauce may be prepared up to this point and completed when chicken is fully baked.)

6. To complete sauce, bring to simmering point. Whisk in just enough cornstarch mixture to lightly thicken. Arrange chicken on warm serving platter. Garnish with orange slices and watercress. Dribble with 2 tablespoons sauce; serve remaining sauce in gravy-boat.

Yield: **Serves 4**

Serving suggestion: Cut 4 medium carrots lengthwise into strips and steam. Sprinkle with 1 tablespoon minced coriander or parsley, ¼ teaspoon freshly grated nutmeg, and 2 teaspoons freshly grated Parmesan cheese. Fold in 1 tablespoon Light Choice sour cream or plain low-fat yogurt. Reheat briefly and serve at once.

7
FISH

FLOUNDER FILLETS WITH SHERRY

Transform this innocuous fish into a savory dish with a quality dry sherry (*never* cooking sherry), crisp pepper, and *fresh* lemon juice.

1 ¼ pounds fillet of flounder, cut
　　into 4 serving pieces
Zest from ½ lemon, chopped
¼ teaspoon salt
2 tablespoons unbleached flour
¼ teaspoon dried thyme
⅛ teaspoon cayenne pepper
1 tablespoon Italian olive oil

2 tablespoons Vegetable Mix (page
　　18)
1 small sweet red pepper, seeded,
　　cut into ¼-inch strips
⅔ cup dry sherry
Minced parsley or fresh coriander
Lemon wedges

1. Wash fish and pat dry. Squeeze lemon juice into a bowl. Add half the salt and beat with a fork to blend. Add fillets, turning several times to coat. Marinate at room temperature for 30 minutes, or cover and refrigerate for up to 1 ½ hours.
2. In a cup, combine flour, lemon zest, remaining salt, thyme, and cayenne pepper. Sprinkle onto a sheet of wax paper. Drain fish by running fillets through forefinger and thumb, compressing fish with fingers. Dip each piece into mixture, lightly coating on both sides.
3. Spread oil evenly over a large nonstick skillet. Heat until hot. Strew Vegetable Mix across skillet; cook for 30 seconds. Arrange fillets on top of mix in one layer. Over medium-high heat, brown fish lightly on one side (about 3 minutes). Turn carefully. Arrange green pepper around fish. Sauté for 2 minutes without disturbing fillets.
4. Pour ¼ cup sherry around sides of skillet. Spoon over fish. Cover and cook for 1 minute. Pour remaining sherry around sides of skillet. Baste fillets several times with juices. Cook, uncovered, until all liquid evaporates.
5. Transfer fish and vegetables to 4 warmed serving plates. Sprinkle with parsley, garnish with lemon wedges, and serve at once.

Yield: **Serves 4**

SHRIMP AND SCALLOPS IN SAFFRON SAUCE

This is a beautiful dish for eye and palate, yet so easy to make. Marinate shrimps and scallops in saffron, herbs, and seasonings, prepare a one-step sauce, then combine the seafood and sauce with bright-green snow peas. It's the saffron that gives it that four-star-restaurant touch.

4 ounces fresh snow peas
1/2 teaspoon whole saffron
2 tablespoons boiling water
2 tablespoons Italian olive oil
1/4 cup fresh lemon juice
1 tablespoon each minced garlic
    and shallot
1/4 teaspoon salt
3/4 teaspoon sugar
1/4 teaspoon powdered thyme
3/4 pound medium-size shrimp,

shelled, deveined, and well
dried
1/2 pound bay scallops, rinsed and
    well dried, each cut in half
1/2 cup Fish Stock (page 21) or a
    combination of Fish Stock
    and Chicken Stock (page 19)
2 tablespoons finely minced parsley
1/4 cup light cream
1 1/2 tablespoons cornstarch

1. Drop snow peas into a saucepan with rapidly boiling water. Cook for 30 seconds. Immediately drain in colander and rinse under cold running water until completely cooled. Gently snap and discard coarse stubble at one end, pulling string down to bottom of each snow pea.

2. Place saffron in the tiniest cup you can find. (I collect hotel breakfast-size jelly jars for this purpose.) Add boiling water. Let stand for 10 minutes. Set aside.

3. Pour 1 tablespoon oil, lemon juice, garlic, shallot, half the salt, sugar, and thyme into a small bowl. Add saffron-water mixture and blend with fork. Combine shrimp and scallops with mixture, turning with spoon several times to coat. Let marinate for 1 hour at room temperature.

4. In a small saucepan, heat 1/3 cup stock with remaining salt and parsley. Bring to simmering point. Add cream and continue cooking just under simmering point for 2 minutes.

5. While sauce slow-cooks, heat remaining 1 tablespoon oil in large nonstick skillet until hot. Lift shrimp and scallops out of marinade and drain. Pour marinade into simmering sauce. Sauté shrimp and

scallops over medium heat until shrimp turn pink and scallops give up their raw look, dribbling up to 2 tablespoons exuded cooking liquid into the saucepan as it accumulates (total cooking time should be 3 to 4 minutes). Remove from heat.

6. Add sauce and snow peas to skillet, stirring to combine. Return skillet to low heat. In a cup, stir enough cornstarch into remaining stock, a little at a time, until sauce is thickness of light cream. Pour half around sides of skillet and cook briefly while stirring for 1 minute. Serve at once.

Yield: **Serves 4**

Serving suggestion: Delightful over crisp "Oven-Baked" Potato Pancakes (page 48).

Notes:

1. Frozen Chinese pea pods, already trimmed, may be substituted for fresh snow peas. Blanch contents of 6-ounce box as in Step 1. Use two-thirds, and refrigerate remainder for another recipe.

2. The size of the shrimp will determine cooking time. I find that medium-size shrimp (about 30 to a pound) are the most tender for this dish, and also cook rapidly.

RED SNAPPER CREOLE

The fish is marinated briefly, coated with Breading Mix to seal in its precious juices, then rapidly sautéed and dressed with a robust tomato-accented sauce to complement its mild, elegant flavor.

For the sauce:

1 10-ounce box whole frozen okra
1 tablespoon white vinegar
1 teaspoon each Italian olive oil
    and sweet butter/margarine
    blend

2 tablespoons finely minced boiled
    ham
2 cups Tomato Sauce (page 23)
1 tablespoon fresh lemon juice

For the fish:

1/4 cup fresh lemon juice
1/4 teaspoon salt
1 1/4 pounds fillets of red snapper
3 tablespoons Breading Mix (page
    17)
1 teaspoon each Italian olive oil

and sweet butter/margarine
    blend
1/2 lemon
Minced parsley
Lemon slices

1. Bring a small saucepan of water to a rolling boil. Add okra and vinegar. Bring to a boil again. Cook, uncovered, over high heat for 2 minutes. Drain in colander. Rinse under cold running water until okra cools. Let drain completely. Cut into 1/4-inch rounds. Set aside.
2. Heat oil and shortening in large nonstick skillet. Over moderate heat, sauté ham with drained okra for 3 minutes. Add Tomato Sauce. Bring mixture to simmering point. Cover and cook gently for 8 minutes. Stir in lemon juice. Pour into saucepan and set aside. Rinse out skillet and dry.
3. To prepare fish, combine lemon juice and salt in a bowl. Add fillets, turning several times to coat. Let stand for 10 minutes. Drain off liquid by running fillets through forefinger and thumb, compressing fish with fingers. Sprinkle Breading Mix across a sheet of wax paper. Dip fish into mix, pressing on both sides to adhere; gently shake off excess.
4. Heat oil and shortening in skillet until hot. Arrange fillets in one layer. Sauté on each side for 3 to 4 minutes. Sprinkle with lemon juice.
5. Arrange fish on warm individual serving plates. Spoon a tablespoon of sauce over each serving, and ladle proportional amounts around fillets. Sprinkle with lemon juice, then minced parsley. Garnish with lemon slices.

Yield: **Serves 4**

CURRIED HALIBUT FILLETS

Eastern halibut and salmon share top ranking on my list of preferred fish. I like halibut for its neutral flavor, which allows me to infuse it with all sorts of stocks and marinades.

1 tablespoon Vegetable Mix (page 18)
¼ cup red wine vinegar
1½ cups Fish Stock (page 21)
1½ teaspoons mild curry powder
¼ teaspoon salt
1 tablespoon minced parsley
4 teaspoons sweet butter/margarine

blend
3 tablespoons unbleached flour
1 tablespoon unsalted tomato paste
⅛ teaspoon cayenne pepper
1 pound fresh halibut fillets, ½-inch thick
1 teaspoon Italian olive oil
Lemon slices

1. In small heavy-bottomed saucepan, combine Vegetable Mix and vinegar. Place over moderate heat and cook, uncovered, until all liquid evaporates. Stir in stock, 1 teaspoon curry powder, ⅛ teaspoon salt, and parsley. When mixture boils, reduce heat to simmering and cook, uncovered, until reduced to 1 cup (about 8 minutes). Strain into bowl, pressing out juices. Rinse out saucepan and dry.
2. Heat 2 teaspoons shortening in saucepan until melted. Add 1 tablespoon flour. Stir and cook for 1 minute. Gradually whisk in strained sauce. Blend in tomato paste and cayenne pepper. Cook over moderate heat until thickened and smooth, whisking often. Remove from heat. Cover to keep warm.
3. Rinse fish; paper-dry. Sprinkle remaining flour, curry powder, and salt onto sheet of wax paper. Dredge fish in mixture.
4. Heat remaining shortening and oil in large nonstick skillet until hot. Arrange fish in one layer and sauté for 3 minutes on each side. Fish should be lightly browned.
5. Reheat sauce briefly, if necessary. Spoon a tablespoon in centers of four warmed individual serving plates. Cover with a portion of fish. Then spoon remaining sauce around fish. Garnish with lemon slices and serve at once.

Yield: **Serves 4**

Serving suggestion: Steam 1 cup of ½-inch cubed and peeled white turnip and 1 cup of shelled peas until tender. Season with ¼ teaspoon freshly grated nutmeg, a pinch of salt, 1 tablespoon minced fresh coriander, and a teaspoon of sweet butter/margarine blend. Sprinkle with 2 teaspoons freshly grated Parmesan cheese and black pepper. Arrange in a circle around fish.

SHRIMP-FILLED CREPES

America's favorite seafood deserves to be glorified. So here is a beautiful party dish. Daintily spiced shrimp and Bosc pear are enveloped in elegantly thin crepes and napped with a creamy, sherry-enriched sauce.

For the sauce:

1¼ cups each Fish Stock (page 21) and Chicken Stock (page 19)

2 tablespoons dry sherry

¼ teaspoon each dried thyme leaves and ground cardamom

2 dashes cayenne pepper

1 tablespoon minced fresh coriander

2 tablespoons light cream or milk

1 tablespoon cornstarch

For the filling and crepes:

1 pound medium shrimp, shelled, deveined, and well dried on paper toweling

4½ teaspoons cornstarch

¼ teaspoon salt

½ teaspoon ground ginger

¼ teaspoon each ground cardamom and dried thyme leaves

2 teaspoons each sweet butter/margarine blend and Italian olive oil

3 tablespoons each minced celery and shallot

1 large firm Bosc pear, peeled, cored, cut into ¼-inch cubes

1 tablespoon dry sherry

2 tablespoons milk or light cream, or a combination of both

2 tablespoons minced fresh coriander

1 recipe Crepes (page 65; see Note below), warmed

1. Prepare sauce first. Put stocks in medium heavy-bottomed saucepan. Over fairly high heat, reduce to 2¼ cups. Measure out 1 cup for filling and set aside. To remaining stocks, add sherry, seasonings, and coriander. Bring to simmering point and cook for 2 minutes. Remove from heat.

2. To prepare the filling, cut each shrimp lengthwise, then crosswise into 4 pieces. Place in bowl. In a cup, combine cornstarch with seasonings. Sprinkle mixture over shrimp, stirring to coat all over. Set aside.

3. In a large nonstick skillet, heat shortening and oil. Over moderate heat, sauté celery and shallot until wilted. Raise heat slightly. Strew

shrimp over mixture, separating pieces. Sauté for 2 minutes more, turning continually. Combine pear with mix and sauté for 1 minute.
4. Pour in sherry. Cook for 30 seconds. Add about ¾ cup reserved stock mixture, a little at a time, stirring continually until liquid becomes moderately thick. Add milk and coriander.
5. To complete recipe for sauce, re-warm over low heat. Whisk in cream or milk. Measure cornstarch into a cup. Gradually add 2 table-spoons of sauce to the cup, blending until smooth with small spoon (or chopstick, which is ideal for this chore). Pour back into warm sauce. Whisk and cook over moderate heat until thickened and smooth.
6. To assemble, place 2 warm crepes on 4 individual serving plates. Evenly distribute filling in center of each crepe. Flip over parallel sides to make a "package." Spoon with hot sauce, and serve at once.

Yield: **Serves 4 as a main course; 8 as a first course**

Note: Crepes may be made a day ahead and reheated 15 minutes before preparing sauce. Here's how: Roll crepes up loosely and place on lightly oiled baking pan. Cover with foil and bake in a preheated 350-degree oven for 12 minutes. Remove from oven and let stand, covered, until ready to fill. Unroll at the beginning of Step 5, before completing sauce and filling with shrimp mix.

SESAME FISH FILLETS

Here's a new way to enjoy juicy fish fillets. Toast oat bran and sesame seeds in a nonstick skillet, dip fillets into an herbed milk bath, then sauté quickly on a thin bed of minced shallot and ginger. Ready to enjoy in less than 20 minutes, including preparation time!

1 tablespoon unhulled sesame seeds (available in health-food stores)

2 tablespoons each oat bran and fine toasted bread crumbs, preferably homemade

1 1/2 tablespoons freshly grated Parmesan cheese

5 tablespoons milk

1 1/2 teaspoons prepared Dijon mustard, preferably unsalted

1 teaspoon unsalted tomato paste

2 teaspoons fresh lime juice

2 teaspoons dried rosemary, finely crushed

1 to 1 1/4 pounds thin fillet of flounder, lemon or gray sole, cut into 4 serving pieces

1 tablespoon each Italian olive oil and sweet butter/margarine blend

2 tablespoons minced shallot

1/2 teaspoon finely chopped fresh ginger

Lime wedges and crisp watercress sprigs

1. Heat small nonstick skillet. Over moderate heat, toast sesame seeds and oat bran until lightly browned, shaking skillet every 30 seconds (about 3 minutes). Turn into a cup. Add bread crumbs, and cheese, stirring to combine.

2. In a medium bowl, blend milk, mustard, tomato paste, lemon juice, and rosemary.

3. Rinse fillets under cold running water. Paper-dry. Add to milk mixture, turning to coat. Let stand for 5 minutes.

4. Sprinkle half of dry mix across a sheet of wax paper. Drain any excess liquid from fish (there will be very little), and place on top of crumb mix. Sprinkle with remaining dry mix, pressing into fish to adhere.

5. Heat oil and shortening in large nonstick skillet. Spread with shallot and ginger, sautéing without stirring over medium-high heat for 30 seconds. Arrange fillets over shallot/ginger mix and cook for 2 minutes. Shake skillet or gently lift fillets with spatula to shift. Cook for 1 minute longer. Turn carefully. Repeat procedure.

6. Transfer to warmed individual serving plates and garnish with lemon wedges and watercress.

Yield: **Serves 4**

SEA BASS WITH HORSERADISH SAUCE

The pungency of horseradish combines with sea bass's naturally strong flavor in this unusual, sharp-edged entree. Important: Use a freshly opened bottle of horseradish, or grate your own, and mix with a little white vinegar and a sprinkling of salt.

4 fillets of black sea bass (two 1¼-pound fish)
1 tablespoon fresh lemon juice
1½ to 1¾ cups Fish Stock (page 21)
1 thin slice lemon peel
¼ teaspoon each dry mustard and salt
2 teaspoons white wine Worcestershire sauce
⅛ teaspoon dried thyme

½ teaspoon dried dill weed
4 sprigs parsley tied into neat bundle with white cotton thread
About 1 cup loosely packed watercress leaves
2½ to 3 teaspoons prepared white horseradish
2 tablespoons Light Choice sour cream

1. Rinse fish and dry with paper toweling. Run fingers over fillets, and with pliers pull out any remaining bones from each fillet. Lay on plate. Sprinkle with lemon juice, turning to coat. Cover and let stand for 30 minutes.
2. Prepare poaching liquid by pouring 1½ cups stock into large nonstick skillet. Add lemon peel, mustard, salt, Worcestershire sauce, dried herbs, and parsley bundle. Bring to a boil. Reduce heat. Cover and simmer for 5 minutes.
3. Arrange fillets in liquid in one layer. Add enough of remaining stock to barely cover fish. Bring to a boil. Cover partially, reduce heat, and simmer for 8 minutes. Line a warm serving platter with watercress leaves. With slotted spatula, lay fish on watercress. Cover loosely with sheet of wax paper.
4. Turn up heat under skillet. Reduce liquid to ¾ cup. Discard lemon peel and parsley bundle, squeezing out juices. Combine horseradish with sour cream and blend well. Whisk mixture into poaching liquid. Taste to see if you would like more horseradish. Cook for 30 seconds. Ladle sauce over fish and serve at once.

Yield: **Serves 4**

SOPHISTICATED CATFISH

A wonderfully textured fish, long relegated to the deep-fry pan, catfish is here treated lightly—poached in a minted broth and dressed in tender tomatoes, white wine, and mushrooms.

For the fish and poaching broth:

¼ cup coarsely chopped shallot
1 tablespoon minced celery
1 thin slice lemon
6 fresh mint leaves, rinsed
⅛ teaspoon each salt and freshly
    ground black pepper

½ cup Fish Stock (page 21) or
    Vegetable Stock (page 20)
½ cup dry white wine
1 to 1¼ pounds fresh catfish
    fillets, skinned, cut into 4
    serving pieces (see Note)

For the sauce:

½ cup Italian unsalted plum
    tomatoes, coarsely chopped
¼ cup dry white wine
4 medium snow-white fresh
    mushrooms, damp-wiped,
    sliced
20 fresh mint leaves, rinsed and
    chopped (about 2 large

    sprigs)
4½ teaspoons sweet
    butter/margarine blend
½ teaspoon freshly grated nutmeg
⅛ teaspoon salt
1 tablespoon unbleached flour
Reserved poaching broth
1 tablespoon cream or milk

1. Prepare poaching broth by combining all ingredients except fish in nonstick skillet large enough to accommodate fish in one layer. Bring to a boil. Reduce heat to simmering; cover and cook for 10 minutes. (May be prepared up to 1 hour before using.) Set aside.
2. To start preparation of sauce, in medium heavy-bottomed saucepan, combine tomatoes, wine, mushrooms, and mint. Bring to a boil; reduce heat to simmering. Cover and simmer for 10 minutes. Set aside. (May be prepared up to 1 hour before using.)
3. Bring poaching broth to a boil. Lay fish in broth, turning several times to coat. Bring to simmering point again. Cover and cook for 7 minutes. Turn carefully with spatula, basting several times. Recover and poach for 7 or 8 minutes longer. Fish should look opaque and still retain its firm texture. With a slotted spatula, transfer to warm serving plate; cover to keep warm. Strain poaching broth into a measuring cup. There should be ½ cup; if less, add enough stock or wine to bring it up to ½ cup. Set aside.

4. In a small heavy-bottomed saucepan, melt shortening. Add nutmeg and salt. Stir and cook over moderate heat for 1 minute. Whisk in flour. Cook for 1 minute. Stir in prepared tomato mixture and cook until thickened. Gradually add reserved poaching broth, blending until smooth. Pour exuded juices from fish into saucepan and combine. Stir in cream or milk. Spoon over fish and serve at once.

Yield: **Serves 4**

Note: For superior flavor, choose thin fillets cut from small catfish.

SWEET AND SOUR FISH

Oriental cooks are celebrated for their sweet-and-sour dishes, most of which are deep-fried. There's no deep-frying in this version, and the "sweet" in sweet and sour remains even though I substitute mainly fruit juice for the half cup of sugar in the traditional recipe.

For the sauce:

⅔ cup each unsweetened pineapple
     or orange juice and water
⅓ cup cider vinegar
3 tablespoons fresh lemon juice
2 tablespoons sugar
1 teaspoon flavorful honey
¼ cup each coarsely chopped

scallion and sweet red pepper
⅛ teaspoon salt
¼ teaspoon dried cilantro
Dash cayenne pepper
2 tablespoons cornstarch dissolved
     in 2 tablespoons water

For the batter and fish:

1 egg yolk
½ cup each unsweetened pineapple
     or orange juice and water
About ⅔ cup unbleached flour
1½ teaspoons non-aluminum
     baking powder

¼ teaspoon freshly grated nutmeg
1 to 1¼ pounds firm-fleshed
     ¼-inch fish fillets, such as
     flounder or turbot
4 tablespoons peanut oil
Orange slices

1. Prepare sauce first. In medium heavy-bottomed saucepan, combine all ingredients except cornstarch mixture and whisk to blend. Place over high heat. Bring to a boil. Reduce heat to simmering. Cook, uncovered, for 10 minutes. Set aside.
2. To prepare batter, whisk together egg yolk, juices, and water in a medium bowl. Stir in ½ cup flour, baking powder, and nutmeg, increasing the amount of flour if necessary to produce a thick batter. Let stand for 2 minutes, stir.
3. Using 2 large nonstick skillets, heat 2 tablespoons oil in each skillet until very hot. Dip fish pieces into batter, immersing for a second or two, then lifting up and draining excess. Immediately arrange in skillets and cook until crispy and brown (3 to 4 minutes). Turn. Cook on second side until equally brown. With slotted spatula, transfer carefully to paper toweling.
4. Reheat sauce briefly. Stir in cornstarch mixture, a little at a time, using enough to make a lightly thickened sauce. Cook over low heat for 1 minute.

5. Arrange fish on warmed serving platter. Spoon sauce over and around fish. Garnish with orange slices and serve immediately.

Yield: **Serves 4**

Variations:

1. Add 2 tablespoons dry sherry to sauce in Step 1.
2. Add ½ pound shelled and deveined raw shrimp to recipe, dipping them in batter and cooking them in hot skillet for 2 minutes on each side. This variation serves 6, with only ⅙ of an egg yolk per portion!

Serving suggestion: Prepare a platter of cooked rice surrounded by ½-inch cubes of steamed carrots seasoned with freshly grated nutmeg, honey to taste, and minced fresh coriander.

Note: For calorie watchers—in the basic recipe, only half the batter is used.

BAKED SALMON FILLETS WITH ESCAROLE

Escarole can be tough, which is why I dislike it in a salad. Here I've softened its disposition by fine-chopping and sautéing it with leeks, garlic, herbs, and spices. Spiked with mustard and arranged in alternating layers with fillets of salmon, it's a new taste experience.

2 medium leeks (use white part
    and 3 inches below)
2 large cloves garlic
About 3/4 pound escarole, tough
    outer leaves removed, rinsed
    and well dried
1 large ripe tomato, skinned and
    seeded
1 pound fresh salmon fillets,
    3/8-inch thick, cut into 4
    serving pieces
1/4 teaspoon salt
Pinch cayenne pepper
1/2 teaspoon freshly grated nutmeg
1 tablespoon Italian olive oil
1 teaspoon dried tarragon,

    crumbled
1/2 teaspoon mild curry powder
1/2 teaspoon prepared Dijon
    mustard, preferably without
    salt
About 1/2 cup each dry white wine
    and Fish Stock (page 21),
    combined and warmed
1 tablespoon light cream
1 teaspoon cornstarch or arrowroot
    flour
4 tablespoons fresh soft bread
    crumbs
4 teaspoons sweet butter/margarine
    blend

1. Use food processor to fine-chop leeks and garlic. Cut leeks into 1-inch slices; quarter garlic. Process on/off 4 to 5 times. Scrape into a measuring cup. You will need 1 cup.
2. Use tender leaves from escarole, breaking them into uniform pieces. Place in workbowl of food processor and process on/off 7 or 8 times until fine-chopped. Scrape into a measuring cup. You will need 1 1/2 cups. Core tomato, hand-chop coarsely.
3. Rinse fish and paper-dry. Sprinkle with salt, pepper, and 1/4 teaspoon nutmeg. Set aside. Preheat oven to 375 degrees.
4. Heat oil in large nonstick skillet until hot. Sauté leeks, garlic, and escarole over medium-high heat, stirring continuously until volume decreases and vegetables soften. Sprinkle with tarragon, remaining 1/4 teaspoon nutmeg, and curry powder. Stir in mustard. Add tomato and combine. Cook for 1 minute.

5. Using butter/margarine blend, lightly grease an ovenproof casserole large enough to hold fish in one layer, or use 4 gratinée dishes. Spoon sautéed mixture into dish(es). Lay fish fillets on top. Pour just enough wine-stock mix around sides of cooking vessel(s) to barely cover fillets, reserving 1 tablespoon for thickening. Baste fish once with juices in dish(es). Bake in center section of preheated oven for 10 minutes.

6. Using spatula to compress fish, pour off liquid from dish(es) into small saucepan. Stir in cream. Bring to a boil and cook for 1 minute. Dissolve cornstarch in reserved tablespoon of wine-stock mix, stirring until very smooth. Dribble into saucepan. Stir and cook until lightly thickened.

7. Strew bread crumbs over fish. Spoon with sauce; dot with shortening. Place under broiler close to heating element for 1 minute. Serve at once.

Yield: **Serves 4**

SOLE EN PAPILLOTE

During a visit to Czechoslovakia a few years back, we lunched at a modest hotel in Bratislava. With fingers crossed, we ordered dishes cooked in brown paper—behind-the-Iron-Curtain papillotes. We needn't have worried, for the food was superb—succulent, and redolent with spices and herbs.

Here's my version of a fish papillote inspired by that memorable meal.

1 pound lemon sole or red snapper fillets	1 tablespoon sweet butter/margarine blend
½ lemon	1 tablespoon unbleached flour
¼ teaspoon salt	1 teaspoon mild curry powder
¼ cup coarsely chopped shallot	1 teaspoon egg yolk
¼ pound snow-white fresh mushrooms, trimmed, damp-wiped, and thinly sliced	¼ teaspoon black pepper
	16 arugula leaves
2 tablespoons wine vinegar	8 ripe cherry tomatoes, seeded and halved
1¼ cups Fish Stock (page 21)	
2 tablespoons dry sherry	4 tablespoons chopped chives

1. Sprinkle fish with juice from lemon. Let stand for 5 minutes. Blot gently with paper toweling. Sprinkle all over with salt.
2. In heavy-bottomed saucepan, combine shallot, mushrooms, and vinegar. Cover and cook over moderate heat for about 8 minutes. Mushrooms will give up their liquid, which will then evaporate. Transfer to bowl. Rinse out saucepan.
3. Place stock and sherry in saucepan. Reduce over moderately high heat to ¾ cup. In another saucepan, heat shortening until bubbly. Whisk in flour and curry powder. Cook without browning for 1 minute. Gradually whisk in reduced stock mix, cooking until thickened.
4. Spoon egg yolk into a cup. Combine with 3 tablespoons sauce, blending well. Pour back into saucepan. Stir and cook for 1 minute. Then stir in mushroom mix and pepper.
5. Preheat oven to 400 degrees. To assemble papillotes, cut four 12-inch squares of parchment paper (available in hardware and cooking equipment shops). In center of each sheet lay equal amounts of arugula leaves flat. On top of leaves place the following in sequence: 2 pieces fish, 4 tomato halves, and 1 tablespoon chives. Spoon equal amounts of thick sauce over all.

6. For each papillote, fold up 2 edges to meet, taking care that food doesn't spill out from sides. Crease down the edges into a 1-inch fold. Repeat once or twice until secure. Then fold open ends in securely (paper clips can be helpful). Place papillotes in shallow baking pan or dish. Bake in center of preheated oven for 15 minutes. Remove clips, if used, and serve on warmed individual plates in the paper bags.

Yield: **Serves 4**

Serving suggestions: In order not to detract from the delicate flavors of the papillotes, serve a quiet accompaniment such as lightly buttered rice, couscous, or potatoes, and steamed green beans or peas.

Variation: Substitute thin salmon or halibut fillets for the sole.

BRAISED CODFISH STEAKS

Codfish, naturally dry-textured, is rendered succulent by a brief marinating in lemon juice with a soupçon of salt. But the secret of its texture is the subsequent braising in a stock-based vegetable sauce.

⅓ cup firmly packed sun-dried tomatoes

Boiling water

¼ cup fresh lemon juice

¼ teaspoon plus ⅛ teaspoon salt

4 codfish steaks (about 1½ pounds)

3 tablespoons unbleached flour

½ teaspoon mild curry powder

1 tablespoon peanut oil

3 tablespoons Vegetable Mix (page 18)

1 small sweet green pepper, seeded, cut into ¼-inch strips

½ cup each Fish Stock (page 21) and white wine (see Note)

1 teaspoon fennel seed, well crushed

2 tablespoons minced Italian flat parsley

1. Rinse tomatoes. Place in cup. Cover with boiling water and let stand until softened. Squeeze out partially and chop coarsely. Set aside.

2. Combine lemon juice and ¼ teaspoon salt in a bowl, beating with a fork to blend. Add fish, turning several times to coat. Let stand for 15 minutes at room temperature, or cover and refrigerate for several hours. When ready to cook, drain off liquid by running steaks through forefinger and thumb, compressing fish with fingers.

3. In a cup, combine flour with curry powder. Sprinkle across a sheet of wax paper. Dip fish into mix, pressing lightly to adhere; turn and coat other side. Shake off excess. Heat oil in large well-seasoned iron skillet until quite hot. Add fish and brown lightly on each side for 2 minutes, scooping up and turning carefully. Transfer to plate.

4. Add Vegetable Mix and green pepper to skillet. Using a spatula, scrape up any crackles from fish and combine with vegetables. Sauté for 1 minute. Add stock, wine, tomatoes, fennel, and parsley, stirring to combine. Bring to simmering point. Lift fish up carefully and return it to skillet, basting with sauce several times. Bring to simmering point. Cover and cook gently for 12 minutes (cooking time may vary with thickness of steaks). Sprinkle with salt and baste again.

5. Transfer fish to warmed individual serving plates. Cover to keep warm. Turn up heat under skillet and reduce liquid until thick (3 to 4 minutes). Ladle and then spread a teaspoon of sauce over each portion; spoon remainder around fish.

Yield: **Serves 4**

SCROD FISH CAKES

These crunchy-crusted fish cakes are anything but traditional.

1 pound fresh scrod fillet (thick section)
4 tablespoons fresh lemon juice
1/4 teaspoon salt
1 1/4 pounds Idaho potatoes, cut into 1/2-inch cubes
1 tablespoon prepared Dijon mustard
1/4 cup each minced shallot and onion
2 teaspoons Worcestershire sauce
2 dashes cayenne pepper
1/2 teaspoon each freshly grated

nutmeg and mild curry powder
1/4 teaspoon freshly ground white or black pepper
1 egg, lightly beaten
2 tablespoons each minced fresh coriander and chives
1/3 to 1/2 cup Breading Mix (page 17)
1 tablespoon each peanut oil and sweet butter/margarine blend
Crisp chicory leaves
Lemon wedges

1. Rinse fish and paper-dry. In a bowl, combine 2 tablespoons lemon juice and half the salt, beating with a fork to blend. Place fish in a bowl, turning to coat. Marinate 30 minutes. Drain.

2. Cut fish into 2 or 3 pieces to fit steamer. Steam over rapidly boiling water until opaque (8 to 10 minutes). Let cool. Transfer to a bowl. Remove the small curved bones. Flake partially with a fork.

3. Cook potatoes in a saucepan of boiling water to cover until tender but still flaky. Drain and return to saucepan. Dry out over moderate heat, shaking saucepan several times. Transfer to another bowl and mash. Stir in mustard, shallot, onion, Worcestershire sauce, cayenne, spices, pepper, and egg. Fold in fish carefully (do not mash), along with coriander and chives.

4. With moistened hands, shape mixture into 12 balls. Sprinkle 1/3 cup Breading Mix across a sheet of wax paper. Roll balls in mix.

5. Prepare cakes in 2 batches in large nonstick skillet, or in two skillets, using half the shortening and half the oil for each batch. Heat the oil mix until quite hot. Arrange 6 cakes in each batch, flattening to 1/2 inch. Over medium heat, sauté on each side for about 3 1/2 minutes until golden brown.

6. Arrange chicory leaves on 4 warmed individual serving plates. Place 3 cakes on top of each serving. Sprinkle with juice from some lemon wedges; garnish with remaining wedges.

Yield: **Serves 4**

Serving suggestions: Lump Crabmeat Sauce (page 150) or Fresh Horseradish Sauce (page 152) adds a zesty note to these fish cakes.

RISOTTO WITH SHRIMP

Risotto in Italy, where it's a perennial favorite, is made with lots and lots of butter and cheese. Now zooming into popularity in this country, it features a combination of creaminess and chewiness found in no other rice dish. My version keeps the wonderful taste while cutting way down on the fat and cheese. A word of caution: This is one dish you can't walk away from while you're cooking it, not even for a minute. But with your first taste, your vigilance will be richly rewarded.

1 medium sweet red pepper
6 cups combined Chicken Stock
    (page 19) and Fish Stock
    (page 21)
1/2 pound fresh shrimp, shelled and
    deveined, each shrimp cut
    lengthwise, then cut into 6
    pieces
1 tablespoon each Italian olive oil
    and sweet butter/margarine
    blend
1 tablespoon minced garlic
3/4 cup coarsely chopped onion
1/4 cup minced shallot

1 cup Italian short-grain rice
    (Arborio)
1 1/2 tablespoons Savory Seasoning
    (page 15)
3/4 cup dry white wine
2 tablespoons minced flat Italian
    parsley or minced fresh basil
1/4 teaspoon salt
2 light dashes cayenne pepper
1/4 cup fresh Parmesan cheese (see
    Note for Breading Mix, page
    17)
Watercress sprigs

1. Char pepper, following directions in Step 1 for Saffron Rice Salad (page 174). Cut into 1-inch chunks. Place in food blender or processor with 1/2 cup stock and puree until very smooth. Set aside.
2. Heat remaining 5 1/2 cups of stock and keep simmering. Add shrimp and poach for 1 minute. Remove shrimp with slotted spoon and set aside.
3. Heat 1 tablespoon each oil and shortening in heavy-bottomed saucepan (an 8-inch stainless steel pot is ideal for this recipe) until hot. Add garlic, onion, and shallot, and sauté over moderate heat until wilted (2 minutes). Add rice. Sprinkle in half the Savory Seasoning. Cook for 3 minutes, scooping up and stirring every 30 seconds. Mixture will begin to adhere to pot after 2 minutes, after which it should be continually stirred.
4. Pour in wine. Stir and cook until most of liquid evaporates (about 2 minutes). Add 1 cup of stock and parsley or basil. Cook until most

of the liquid is absorbed (about 3 minutes). Add pepper purée. Continue to cook and stir for 3 minutes. While stirring, add remaining stock, a half-cup at a time, allowing liquid to be absorbed before each addition.

5. Gently stir shrimp, salt, pepper, and cheese into rice. Cook for 1 minute over low heat. Arrange on warmed individual plates, garnished with watercress sprigs.

Yield: **Serves 4 as a main course; 8 as a first course**

SKEWERED MONKFISH

Monkfish, called *lotte* or *ange de mer* in France, has recently come into favor in this country. Its meaty texture makes it an excellent choice for skewering and close-to-the-heat broiling. Since its flesh is denser than that of flatfish, cooking time will vary with the performance of your broiler.

¼ cup fresh lemon juice
2 tablespoons red wine vinegar
1 teaspoon dried cilantro, crumbled
⅛ teaspoon each salt and cayenne
*   pepper*
¼ cup coarsely chopped shallots
1 pound fresh monkfish, membrane
*   removed, cut into 1-inch*
*   cubes*
1 large sweet red pepper, seeded,
*   cut into 1-inch pieces*

1 large sweet green pepper, seeded,
*   cut into 1-inch pieces*
8 snow-white fresh mushroom caps,
*   damp-wiped*
2 tablespoons melted sweet
*   butter/margarine blend*
2 tablespoons freshly grated
*   Parmesan cheese*
1 large bunch crisp watercress,
*   tough stems removed, rinsed*
*   and dried*

1. In a medium bowl, combine lemon juice, vinegar, cilantro, salt, and cayenne pepper. Beat with fork to blend. Stir in shallots. Add fish, turning several times to coat. Marinate for 1 hour at room temperature.
2. Drop peppers into pot of boiling water and cook for 2 minutes. Drain.
3. Preheat broiler. Onto each of 8 or more small trussing skewers, thread drained fish chunks alternately with peppers, ending with 1 mushroom cap.
4. Arrange on rack in shallow broiling pan. Brush with melted shortening. Broil 4 inches from source of heat for 6 minutes. Spoon half the marinade onto skewers. Turn. Return to heat and broil for 6 minutes. Turn. Sprinkle with Parmesan cheese and broil for 3 minutes more. Turn once more and broil for 2 minutes.
5. Line 4 warm serving plates with watercress. For each serving, push fish and vegetables carefully off skewers onto watercress and spoon with pan juices.

Yield: **Serves 4**

Serving suggestion: Pasta with Onion/Shallot Sauce (page 64).

8

MEAT

TWO VERY SPECIAL BURGERS

Refreshing departures from the All-American Hamburger. The Barbecue Burger is spiked with jalapeño peppers (take care not to touch your eyes when handling them), and seasoned with my Barbecue Sauce and Dijon mustard. The Mixed Meat Burgers derive their flavor from ground veal and pork. Make them on your outdoor grill or in a well-seasoned iron skillet.

BARBECUE BURGERS

2 teaspoons Italian olive oil
2 teaspoons minced garlic
3 tablespoons minced shallot
2 tablespoons minced jalapeño
    pepper
1 pound lean ground beef
¼ cup Breading Mix (page 17)
¼ teaspoon salt
½ cup Barbecue Sauce (page
    147)
2 teaspoons prepared Dijon
    mustard, preferably without
    salt
2 tablespoons minced fresh
    coriander
1 tablespoon sweet
    butter/margarine blend

1. Heat oil in small nonstick skillet. Over medium heat, sauté garlic, shallot, and pepper for 2 minutes without browning. Turn into a bowl.
2. Add meat, Breading Mix, and salt, blending well. In a cup, combine ¼ cup Barbecue Sauce with mustard and coriander. Stir into meat. Shape into 4 burgers, flattening to desired thickness.
3. Heat shortening in well-seasoned iron skillet until quite hot. Over medium-high heat, brown meat for 2 minutes on each side. Brush with 2 tablespoons reserved Barbecue Sauce. Turn. Brush with remaining 2 tablespoons sauce. Sauté until cooked to your taste.

Yield: **Serves 4**

MIXED MEAT BURGERS

5 teaspoons Italian olive oil
2 tablespoons Vegetable Mix (page 18)
1/4 pound boiled ham
1/2 pound each lean ground veal and pork
1 tablespoon Savory Seasoning (page 15)
Pinch salt
2 tablespoons minced parsley
2 tablespoons freshly grated

Parmesan cheese
1/2 cup loosely packed soft fresh bread crumbs from Sourdough French Bread (page 162), or good-quality commercial French or Italian bread
6 tablespoons red wine
3 tablespoons Chicken Stock (page 19), or canned unsalted Beef Stock
1 tablespoon unsalted tomato paste

1. Heat 2 teaspoons oil in small nonstick skillet. Over medium heat, sauté Vegetable Mix for 1 minute. Add ham and sauté for 1 minute longer. Turn into a bowl. Add meat, seasonings, parsley, and Parmesan, blending well.

2. In a cup, combine bread crumbs and 4 tablespoons wine. Mix with meat and shape into 4 burgers, flattening to desired thickness.

3. In a cup, combine remaining 2 tablespoons wine with stock and tomato paste. Set aside.

4. Heat remaining 3 teaspoons of oil in a well-seasoned iron skillet until quite hot. Over medium-high heat, brown meat on both sides. Pour stock mixture around sides of skillet. When it bubbles up, spoon it over meat. Cook for 1 minute. Turn, baste meat with liquid. Sauté until cooked to your taste.

Yield: **Serves 4**

MEATBALLS STROGANOFF WITH PEPPERS

These meatballs are spiked with tomato paste and Dijon mustard, then basted with red wine and slightly sweet balsamic vinegar.

1 pound extra lean ground beef or veal, or a combination of both
5 tablespoons toasted bread crumbs, preferably homemade
1 1/2 tablespoons Savory Seasoning (page 15)
1 1/2 teaspoons each prepared unsalted Dijon mustard and unsalted tomato paste
3 tablespoons each dry red wine, Chicken Stock (page 19), and milk
1 tablespoon unbleached flour

4 teaspoons Italian olive oil
2 tablespoons minced shallot
2 teaspoons minced fresh ginger
1 large sweet green pepper, seeded, cut into 1/4-inch strips
2 tablespoons balsamic vinegar
1/2 cup each Chicken Stock and dry red wine
2 tablespoons minced parsley
1/4 teaspoon salt
1/4 cup each Light Choice sour cream and plain low-fat yogurt
1/2 teaspoon freshly grated nutmeg

1. In a small bowl, combine meat with bread crumbs and Savory Seasoning, blending well. In a cup, combine mustard, tomato paste, wine, stock, and milk, beating with fork to blend. Pour into meat mixture and combine. Let stand for 5 minutes. Shape into 20 balls. Roll balls in flour, shaking off excess.

2. Heat 3 teaspoons oil in large nonstick skillet until very hot. Add balls. Over medium-high heat, sauté until brown, rolling when necessary to brown evenly (about 5 minutes). Transfer to plate. Pour off fat from skillet.

3. Add remaining 1 teaspoon oil to skillet. Sauté shallot, ginger, and pepper over medium heat until wilted but not brown. Stir in vinegar and cook for 1 minute. Add stock and wine. Bring to a boil. Return browned meat to skillet, gently spooning with sauce. Reduce heat to simmering. Cover and cook for 25 minutes.

4. Stir in parsley and salt. Raise heat. Slow-boil, basting meat often, until liquid is reduced by half (about 5 minutes). Stir in sour cream and yogurt; sprinkle with nutmeg. Cook, just under boiling point, until heated through (about 3 minutes). Serve at once on warmed individual plates.

Yield: **Serves 4**

CARAWAY MEATBALLS

Beef and veal are combined here with caraway, ground nuts, a touch of ham, and special seasonings. Serve as a main course or pierced with cocktail picks as an hors d'oeuvre.

For the meat:

1/3 cup firmly packed soft rye bread
   crumbs
1 teaspoon balsamic vinegar
1/4 cup Chicken Stock (page 19)
1 teaspoon fresh lemon juice
1 teaspoon partially crushed
   caraway seed
1/2 teaspoon each cumin and mild

   curry powder
1/4 cup pulverized walnuts
1/2 pound each lean ground beef
   and veal
2 tablespoons minced boiled ham
2 tablespoons finely minced fresh
   coriander
4 teaspoons Italian olive oil

For the sauce:

2 teaspoons Italian olive oil
2 tablespoons seeded and chopped
   jalapeño peppers
1/3 cup minced onion
1/4 pound snow-white fresh
   mushrooms, ends trimmed,

   damp-wiped, coarsely chopped
3/4 cup Chicken Stock (page 19)
2 tablespoons fresh lemon juice
1 tablespoon minced fresh coriander
1/4 teaspoon salt

1. Place bread crumbs in a measuring cup. Stir in vinegar, stock, and lemon juice. Combine mixture with caraway seed, spices, and walnuts.

2. Put beef and veal in bowl. Combine with ham, bread mixture, and coriander. Shape into 20 1½-inch balls. Heat oil over medium-high heat in large nonstick skillet. Brown balls all over, shaking skillet often to assist in rolling.

3. While meat browns, prepare cooking sauce. In medium heavy-bottomed saucepan, heat oil. When hot, add peppers, onion, and mushrooms. Sauté over medium-high heat until lightly browned (about 5 minutes). Stir in stock, lemon juice, coriander, and salt. Bring to a simmering point. Nestle browned meatballs in center of skillet; pour sauce around sides of skillet. Combine gently. Lower heat to simmering. Cover and cook for 25 minutes, basting and turning balls once midway.

4. Uncover. Turn up heat and reduce sauce until it becomes syrupy, stirring carefully to prevent sticking.

Yield: **Serves 4 to 5**

SAUTÉED STEAK WITH ONION MARMALADE

I discovered this innovative condiment in one of San Francisco's elegant restaurants concealed under slices of cooked meat or poultry. Here is a soft pillow of orange-tinged onion marmalade for steak with red wine sauce.

2²/₃ cups Chicken Stock (page 19), or canned unsalted beef stock
2¹/₂ cups coarsely chopped onion
¹/₄ cup coarsely chopped shallot
¹/₄ teaspoon each salt and freshly grated nutmeg
Dash cayenne pepper
1 teaspoon finely chopped orange zest
2 tablespoons wine vinegar
4 1-inch thick sirloin or filet mignon steaks, well trimmed (1¹/₄ pounds)

¹/₂ teaspoon each mild curry powder, chili con carne seasoning, and crushed dried rosemary, or 2 teaspoons Savory Seasoning (page 15)
2 teaspoons each Italian olive oil and sweet butter/margarine blend
¹/₄ cup fruity red wine (such as Zinfandel)
1 tablespoon Light Choice sour cream
Watercress sprigs

1. In a medium heavy-bottomed saucepan, combine 2 cups stock, onion, shallot, half the salt, half the seasonings, orange zest, and vinegar. Bring to a boil. Cook, uncovered, over medium-high heat until all liquid evaporates (20 to 25 minutes), stirring often toward end of cooking time. Cover and remove from heat.

2. Paper-wipe steaks. Sprinkle and rub with remaining salt and seasonings. Heat oil and 1 teaspoon shortening in large well-seasoned iron skillet until hot. Over medium-high heat, sauté steaks on each side for 4 to 5 minutes (medium-rare). Transfer to warm plate. Cover loosely with wax paper. Pour off any liquid remaining in skillet.

3. Add wine to skillet. Over medium heat, deglaze by scraping up bits with spatula. Add remaining ²/₃ cup stock. Bring to a boil and over high heat reduce to ¹/₄ cup. Swirl in remaining 1 teaspoon shortening.

4. Reheat marmalade briefly. Stir in sour cream. Spoon equal portions on warmed individual serving plates. Arrange steak on plates. Pour exuded steak juices into skillet. Stir, then ladle sauce over meat. Serve at once, garnished with watercress.

Yield: **Serves 4**

BEEF IN RED WINE

Lean beef, marinated in a medley of red wine, rice wine vinegar, and fruit juice concentrate, then accented with spices and garlic, makes a dish burnished with a deep-brown gravy and old-fashioned flavor.

For the marinade:

2 1/2 cups dry red wine
1/4 cup frozen orange juice
   concentrate
1 large onion, coarsely chopped

2 tablespoons Savory Seasoning
   (page 15)
1/4 cup rice wine vinegar
6 whole cloves, crushed

For the meat and sauce:

1 1 1/2-inch-thick slice beef round
   (about 3 pounds)
3 tablespoons unbleached flour
1/4 teaspoon each ground allspice,
   cumin, and mild curry
   powder
2 tablespoons Italian olive oil
1 1/2 cups well-washed, coarsely
   chopped leek, including tender
   green section
8 large cloves garlic, peeled and

   quartered
3 tablespoons unsalted tomato paste
About 1 1/2 cups Chicken Stock
   (page 19) or water
1 Bouquet Garni (page 16)
1 to 1 1/4 cups Tomato Sauce
   (page 23)
1/4 teaspoon salt (optional)
Freshly ground black pepper
Orange slices

1. To prepare marinade, combine 2 cups wine and remaining ingredients in fairly narrow non-aluminum bowl (a 1 3/4-quart Corning Ware bowl with cover is excellent). Cut meat into 2 pieces; pierce all over with sharp-pronged fork. Place in marinade, turning several times to coat. Cover and refrigerate overnight, turning once or twice. Drain meat, pushing off onions. Pat dry with paper toweling. Strain marinade into bowl, pressing out juices and reserving. Discard solids.

2. Preheat oven to 375 degrees. In a cup, combine flour with spices. Sprinkle half across a sheet of wax paper. Lay meat over it and sprinkle with remaining mixture, pressing to adhere. Shake off excess.

3. Heat 1 1/2 tablespoons oil in heavy enameled Dutch oven until hot. Over medium-high heat, brown meat on each side for 2 1/2 to 3 minutes, turning carefully with metal spatula. Transfer to plate. Add remaining ½ tablespoon oil to pot. Sauté leek and garlic until lightly brown, scraping up cracklings from meat.

4. Remove half the sautéed mix from pot; spread out remainder. Lay browned meat on mixture in one layer. Strew balance of mix over meat. In a saucepan, combine remaining ½ cup wine with reserved marinade, tomato paste, and stock or water. Bring to a slow boil and cook for 3 minutes. Pour around meat. Drop in Bouquet Garni. Bring to simmering point. Cover and simmer on top of the stove for 3 minutes. Transfer to center section of oven. Bake for 40 minutes. Uncover and turn meat carefully.

5. Reduce oven heat to 350 degrees. Re-cover and bake until fork-tender (1¼ to 1½ hours), turning meat twice at equal intervals. Sauce will be reduced and very thick. Remove from oven and uncover partially. Let stand for 15 minutes.

6. Discard Bouquet Garni after pressing out juices. Drain meat and transfer to carving board. With very sharp knife, cut into ¼-inch slices. Transfer slices to large nonstick skillet and cover.

7. Place Dutch oven over low heat on top of stove. Add enough Tomato Sauce to make a thick, pourable gravy. Taste for salt, adding it if desired. Stir in pepper. Cook over moderate heat for 2 minutes, stirring continually. Pour sauce over meat. Cover and let stand for 30 minutes so that flavors are absorbed.

8. Re-warm over very low heat. Arrange on hot platter, garnished with orange slices.

Yield: **6 or more servings**

Note: Store any leftovers in boilable pouches and freeze. When re-heated in a pot of boiling water, the meat is exceptionally tender.

Serving suggestions: Buckwheat Spätzle (page 66) or Sautéed Polenta (page 62) go nicely with this entree.

VEAL FLORENTINE

In this contemporary version of an Italian classic, spinach is blanketed with thin-sliced veal scallops that are quickly sautéed, then sweetened, ever so gently, with a luscious raisin sauce.

1 recipe Raisin Sauce (page 153)
1 10-ounce box frozen leaf spinach, cooked
1 1/2 tablespoons each Italian olive oil and sweet butter/margarine blend, combined
3 tablespoons minced boiled ham

1/2 teaspoon freshly grated nutmeg
1 teaspoon dry tarragon leaves, crumbled
2 tablespoons unbleached flour
1 pound thin-sliced veal scallops, cut from the leg, flattened to 1/8-inch thickness

1. Prepare Raisin Sauce. Cover and set aside.
2. Put cooked spinach in strainer, and press out as much liquid as possible. Transfer to cutting board and fine-chop.
3. Heat a small nonstick skillet with half the shortening until hot. Add ham and cook for 1 minute. Combine with spinach and half the nutmeg. Cover and set aside.
4. In a cup, combine remaining 1/8 teaspoon nutmeg with tarragon and flour. Sprinkle across a sheet of wax paper. Dredge veal in mix, shaking off excess. Using two large nonstick skillets, sauté the meat, using half the shortening in each skillet. Heat the shortening until very hot. Add veal and cook for 1 1/2 minutes on each side.
5. While meat cooks, reheat Raisin Sauce and spinach briefly. Arrange equal portions of spinach on warmed individual serving plates. Cover with meat; spoon with hot sauce.

Yield: **Serves 4**

Serving suggestion: Try these scallops with my Skillet "French-Fried" Potatoes (page 47).

Note: If you prefer to use fresh spinach, use 1 to 1 1/4 pounds unwashed spinach. Break off the leaves from stems. Soak the leaves in a basin of cold water. Lift out of basin and drain water. Refill the basin and soak again. Spinach is fully clean and free of sand when drain water runs clear. Squeeze out as much liquid as possible. Place spinach in a large saucepan. Cover and cook over moderate heat until limp (3 to 4 minutes). Transfer to chinois or strainer and press out liquid. Transfer to cutting board and fine-chop. (May be prepared ahead of time to this point and refrigerated.)

BLANQUETTE OF VEAL WITH FRUIT

Tender braised veal is bathed in a fruity sauce with the heady essence of Madeira wine. Serve it over just-cooked rice, noodles, or pasta.

4 ounces unsulphured dry apricots
    (available in health-food
    stores)
1/2 cup fresh orange juice
1/2 cup Malmsey Madeira
1/2 teaspoon each cinnamon,
    freshly grated nutmeg, and
    dried thyme
2 teaspoons minced garlic
2 tablespoons Italian olive oil
1 1/4 pounds lean stewing veal, cut
    into 1-inch chunks
1 large leek, split and well rinsed,
    cut into 1/4-inch slices

1 medium sweet green pepper,
    seeded, cut into 1/4-inch strips
1/2 cup Chicken Stock (page 19)
4 whole cloves
8 parsley sprigs, tied into neat
    bundle with white cotton
    thread
1 tablespoon arrowroot or
    cornstarch
2 tablespoons milk or cream
Minced fresh coriander or
    just-snipped dill
Orange sections

1. Rinse apricots and dry with paper toweling. Place in a small non-aluminum bowl. Add orange juice and half the Madeira. Set aside.
2. In a bowl, combine seasonings, garlic, and 1 tablespoon oil. Add meat, turning several times until well coated. Cover and let stand for 30 minutes.
3. Heat remaining 1 tablespoon oil in a Dutch oven (preferably enameled). Add leek and green pepper. Sauté over moderate heat for 2 minutes. Add meat. Stir and cook until it loses its pink color (about 5 minutes). Pour remaining half of wine around sides of pot. Combine with meat. Then add stock, apricots (including soaking liquid), cloves, and parsley bundle. Bring to boiling point. Reduce heat to simmering. Cover and simmer until fork-tender (1 1/2 to 2 hours), stirring from time to time and adjusting heat when necessary to keep meat from sticking. (May be prepared up to this point a day ahead, and thickened, if desired, just before serving.)
4. If serving directly after cooking time is completed, put arrowroot or cornstarch into a cup. Slowly stir in milk or cream until mixture is smooth. Dribble into hot sauce and cook until lightly thickened. Transfer to a warm serving bowl. Sprinkle with herbs, and garnish with orange sections.

Yield: **Serves 4**

VEAL AND CHICKEN MOUSSE IN GRAPE LEAVES

A number of ingredients are ground to pâté-like texture to achieve this delicate mousse, which is buoyed to exotic tanginess by thin wrappings of grape leaves. An excellent main course, it is also wonderful for party hors d'oeuvres, because all preparations may be done the day before.

1 8-ounce jar grape leaves packed in brine
1/2 pound each boned and skinned chicken breasts and veal flank
1 teaspoon prepared Dijon mustard, preferably without salt
1/4 cup tightly packed parsley florets
1 teaspoon mild curry powder
10 whole cloves, crushed
1 tablespoon frozen orange juice concentrate
2 tablespoons dry sherry

1 large clove garlic, halved
2 large shallots, quartered
3 tablespoons coarsely chopped boiled ham
1 egg white
1 small unsalted pimento, drained on paper toweling
2 tablespoons Breading Mix (page 17)
1 tablespoon cream or milk
About 1 1/2 tablespoons Italian olive oil
2 cups Tomato Sauce (page 23), heated

1. Pull out one bundle of grape leaves from jar. Unfold and separate. Fill jar of remaining leaves to top with water, cover, and refrigerate for use in another recipe. Rinse each leaf under warm running water. Then drop all leaves in a pot of boiling water and blanch for 1 minute. Lay flat on layers of paper toweling to dry. Roll up paper toweling with leaves and set aside.
2. Fit food processor with steel blade. Cut chicken and veal into 1-inch chunks, removing any membranes (the processor won't grind them). Place in workbowl. Add mustard, parsley, curry powder, cloves, juice, sherry, garlic, and shallots. Process until chicken and veal are well chopped (20 to 30 seconds). Add ham, egg white, pimento, Breading Mix, and cream or milk. Process for 10 seconds. Scrape into a bowl and chill for 15 minutes.
3. To make 14 bundles, start with largest leaves. Fill, shiny sides

down, by placing a heaping tablespoon of mousse in the center of the leaf. Flatten slightly. Overlap two sides over mousse. Fold up other sides to complete the bundle. Place, seam down, in lightly oiled steamer. To use smaller leaves, overlap one on another so that the two leaves together are about the same size as one large leaf. Then follow preceding instructions.

4. Brush bundles with oil. Cover tightly and steam for 25 minutes. Transfer in layers to storage bowl. Pour Tomato Sauce over all. Let cool. Cover and refrigerate for at least 4 hours (or overnight) to permit flavors to permeate bundles.

5. To serve, slowly reheat in nonstick saucepan or skillet, spooning with sauce from time to time. Transfer to a warmed serving bowl and serve very hot as a main course.

Yield: **14 bundles**

Variations:

1. To serve as hors d'oeuvres, set out 28 to 30 leaves. Mound each leaf with 2 teaspoons mousse; *do not flatten.* Continue with balance of recipe. After reheating bundles in sauce (Step 5), pierce with cocktail picks and serve hot.

2. Breading Mix offers a concentrated flavor boost. If you don't have it on hand, substitute 2 tablespoons fine toasted bread crumbs and 1 ½ teaspoons freshly grated Parmesan cheese.

VEAL SHANK WITH CRANBERRY SAUCE

Wet-clay cooking, millennia old, is four-star modern. It's a time/labor saver: Once in the clay pot, the food needs no attention. It's healthful, too, since all the nutrients are locked in and only a tiny amount of fat is required.

2 tablespoons each unbleached flour and stone-ground yellow cornmeal

1/4 teaspoon salt

1 teaspoon dried mint

6 1/2-inch slices veal shank (about 1 3/4 pounds)

2 tablespoons Italian olive oil

2 teaspoons minced garlic

1 large onion, thinly sliced

3 large snow-white fresh mushrooms, ends trimmed, damp-wiped, coarsely chopped

1 1/2 cups finely shredded Savoy cabbage

1/2 cup fresh cranberries, rinsed

1/2 cup unsweetened apple juice

2 tablespoons minced parsley

1/2 cup dry white wine

3/4 cup Ancini pasta

1. Soak clay pot (including cover) in tepid water for 20 to 30 minutes.
2. In a cup, combine flour, cornmeal, salt, and mint. Sprinkle half across a sheet of wax paper. Damp-wipe veal, then rub dry with paper toweling. Lay slices on dry mixture, pressing to adhere. Sprinkle with remaining mix, pressing into meat. Shake off excess.
3. Heat 1 tablespoon oil in large well-seasoned iron skillet. Add 3 meat slices and brown lightly on both sides over medium-high heat. Transfer to a plate. Using remaining oil heated in skillet, repeat procedure for the other 3 slices.
4. To a skillet, add garlic, onion, and mushrooms. Sauté for 3 minutes, stirring continually. Add cabbage and sauté for 1 minute more. Add cranberries, apple juice, and parsley. Bring to a boil.
5. Empty clay pot (do not dry). Spread half of mixture across ridged bottom section. Arrange meat on top. Spoon remaining mixture over meat. Pour wine around sides of pot. Cover tightly. Position oven rack in bottom third of oven. Set thermostat at 375 degrees. Place pot on rack and bake for 1 hour and 5 minutes.
6. Ten minutes before meat is done, bring a pot of water to a rolling boil. Add ancini (a pebble-shaped pasta) and cook to desired texture (I prefer to cook it for 10 minutes). Drain well.
7. Uncover clay pot, keeping your head back from the steam. Arrange meat on warmed individual plates along with a portion of pasta. Serve equal amounts of thick vegetable sauce over pasta, leaving spoonfuls to spread across each slice of meat.

Yield: **Serves 4 to 5**

VEAL CHOPS PAPRIKASH

It's the paprika that gives this dish its distinctive Hungarian flavor. But don't let the fiery redness of the spice fool you—not all paprikas are torrid, some are mild. I use the mild version to make a spicy yet mellow sauce for tender veal chops.

4 teaspoons mild paprika (see Note)
1/4 teaspoon salt
2 teaspoons minced garlic
4 loin or rib veal chops, cut 1/2-inch thick (about 1 1/2 pounds)
2 tablespoons Italian olive oil
1/2 cup coarsely chopped onion
1/4 cup coarsely chopped sweet red pepper
2 cups peeled 1/2-inch cubes butternut squash
1/2 cup dry sherry
1/2 cup Chicken Stock (page 19)
2 tablespoons frozen orange juice concentrate
1 Bouquet Garni (page 16)
2 teaspoons stone-ground yellow cornmeal
3 tablespoons Light Choice sour cream, or plain low-fat yogurt
Freshly ground black pepper

1. In a cup, combine 2 teaspoons paprika with salt and garlic, stirring until well blended. Damp-wipe chops, then rub all over with mixture. Wrap in freezer paper and refrigerate for several hours or overnight.
2. Spread half the oil across a large well-seasoned iron skillet and heat until hot. Sauté chops on each side until lightly browned (5 to 6 minutes). Transfer to plate. Cover to keep warm.
3. Add remaining oil to skillet. Sauté onion, red pepper, and squash for 3 minutes, stirring often. Pour in sherry and stock. Bring to a boil. Stir in concentrate and remaining 2 teaspoons paprika. Drop in bouquet garni. Bring to simmering point. Return browned chops to skillet, turning several times to coat. Cover and cook until tender (about 45 minutes), turning once and spooning with sauce. Transfer chops to warm serving plate; cover to keep warm. Raise heat under skillet. Cook sauce over medium-high heat for 5 minutes. Discard bouquet garni after pressing out juices.
4. Measure cornmeal into a small cup. Add 2 tablespoons hot gravy and stir to blend. While stirring, dribble mixture into skillet. Cook over medium-high heat until sauce thickens and is reduced by half.
5. Return chops to skillet, turning to coat. Cover and simmer for 5 minutes. Stir in sour cream or yogurt and heat until just under simmering point. Arrange chops on warmed serving plates, surrounded by thick sauce and sprinkled with pepper to taste.

Yield: **Serves 4**

Note: For superior flavor, use a freshly opened container of paprika.

VEAL ROULADE WITH CHICKEN MOUSSE

This is a house special of ours for an intimate dinner party. Making this multi-textured and -flavored entree does take a bit of doing, but the mousse can be prepared a day ahead and the dish can be finished an hour or two before serving.

For the mousse:

1/4 cup wild rice, rinsed
1/2 cup water
1/2 cup Chicken Stock (page 19)
2 tablespoons Italian olive oil
4 teaspoons minced garlic
1/2 cup finely chopped onion
2 tablespoons seeded and finely chopped jalapeño peppers

1 small whole boned and skinned chicken breast (about 10 ounces)
3 teaspoons Savory Seasoning (page 15)
3 parsley florets
1 teaspoon egg yolk
2 tablespoons cream

For the meat and sauce:

4 large 1/4-inch slices veal scallops, cut from the leg (1 pound), flattened to 1/8-inch thickness
1 tablespoon unbleached flour
1/4 pound snow-white fresh mushrooms, damp-wiped and thinly sliced
1/2 cup fruity red wine (such as

Zinfandel)
1/4 cup Chicken Stock, room temperature
2 tablespoons unsalted tomato paste
4 sprigs parsley tied into neat bundle with white cotton thread
2 tablespoons fresh lemon juice
Orange slices, decoratively cut

1. In small heavy-bottomed saucepan, soak rice in water for 1 hour. Add stock. Bring to a boil. Reduce heat to simmering. Cover and cook for 35 to 40 minutes, stirring twice at equal intervals. Finished rice should be tender yet retain its firm texture (most of the liquid will be absorbed). Uncover and set aside.

2. Heat 1 tablespoon oil over moderate heat in small nonstick skillet. Briefly sauté half of the garlic, half of the onion, and half of the peppers until wilted but not brown (about 2 minutes). Let stand in skillet.

3. Cut away and discard the string of white cartilage from chicken and slice into 2-inch chunks. Fit food processor with steel blade. To workbowl add chicken, 1 teaspoon Savory Seasoning, parsley florets, egg yolk, and cream. Process for 20 seconds. Scrape mixture into small bowl. (Mousse may be prepared a day ahead up to this point and refrigerated.) Drain any liquid from rice. Fold into mousse until well combined (there should be about 2 cups).

4. Damp-wipe veal. Cut each slice in half and rub all over with remaining 2 teaspoons Savory Seasoning. Mound 1 heaping tablespoon of mousse in center of 4 slices of meat. Cover with remaining 4 slices of meat. Secure edges with toothpicks. Shape remaining mousse into 4 balls.

5. Sprinkle flour across a sheet of wax paper. Dip each roulade and mousse ball into flour, gently rubbing with fingers to evenly distribute. Tap off excess.

6. Heat remaining 1 tablespoon oil in well-seasoned iron skillet until moderately hot. Add roulades and mousse balls. Sauté for 1½ minutes on each side. Strew remaining uncooked garlic, onion, and peppers around meat; add mushrooms. Sauté for 2 minutes.

7. In a measuring cup, blend wine with stock and tomato paste. Pour around sides of skillet and cook for 1 minute. Drop in parsley bundle, pushing into liquid. Spoon sauce over meat and mousse. Bring to simmering point. Cover tightly and cook for 1 hour, turning with spatula and spooning lightly thickened sauce over meat/mousse every 15 minutes. Uncover; spoon on sauce. Re-cover and let stand for 10 minutes. Transfer roulades and mousse to a serving plate. Pull toothpicks out carefully. Cover to keep warm.

8. Add lemon juice to sauce. Cook over moderate heat for 1 minute. Discard parsley bundle after pressing out juices. Ladle sauce over roulades and mousse. Garnish with orange slices and serve at once.

Yield: **4 large servings**

Variation: Chicken Mousse Hors d'Oeuvre: Add 1 teaspoon Savory Seasoning to mixture. Flatten a heaping tablespoon of mousse into ¼-inch patties and sauté in batches on both sides in large nonstick skillet that has been brushed with 1 teaspoon oil per batch. Serve hot, sprinkled with fresh lemon juice. Serve on Oat Crackers (page 155) or with forks.

SAVORY LAMB STEW OVER CORNBREAD POINTS

Exotically spiced lamb stew, blanketed in a smooth Madeira sauce, adorns Dinner Cornbread.

½ boned leg of lamb, shank end
　　(about 2½ pounds), trimmed
　　of all visible fat, gristle, and
　　membranes, plus 1 medium
　　lamb bone
½ teaspoon each allspice and
　　dried mint leaves
1 teaspoon dried rubbed sage leaves
2½ tablespoons unbleached flour
1½ tablespoons each Italian olive
　　oil and sweet
　　butter/margarine blend
1 cup coarsely chopped onion
⅓ cup coarsely chopped shallot
1 medium sweet green pepper,
　　seeded, cut into ¼-inch strips

2 medium turnips, peeled, cut into
　　½-inch cubes
2 large ripe tomatoes, cored,
　　seeded, skinned, cut into
　　1-inch chunks
½ cup Malmsey Madeira
1 cup Chicken Stock (page 19)
1 Bouquet Garni (page 16),
　　including 2 tablespoons
　　partially crushed juniper
　　berries (see Note)
¼ teaspoon salt (optional)
1 recipe Dinner Cornbread,
　　warmed (page 166)
Minced parsley

1. Damp-wipe meat; cut into 1-inch chunks. In a cup, combine and blend allspice and herbs with flour. Spread meat across large sheet of wax paper; add bone. Sprinkle with mix, using fingers to assist in coating evenly.
2. Heat 1 tablespoon each oil and shortening in heavy enameled Dutch oven until quite hot. Add meat and bone, separating pieces and spreading across pot. Sauté over medium-high heat until meat is lightly crusted, turning often with spatula (about 8 minutes). Transfer all ingredients to bowl. Pour off any fat.
3. Add remaining oil and shortening to skillet. When hot, sauté onion and shallot over medium-high heat, scraping up crusty residue from meat. Cook over medium-high heat for 2 minutes. Add green pepper and turnips. Sauté for 2 minutes. Combine tomatoes with mixture. Cook for 2 minutes more.
4. Push ingredients to center of skillet. Pour wine around sides of pot.

Cook for 1 minute without stirring. Then pour in stock. Bring to a boil, stirring to combine. Return browned meat and bone to Dutch oven. Drop in Bouquet Garni, pushing it into liquid. Preheat oven to 325 degrees.

5. Reduce heat under Dutch oven. Cover and simmer for 10 minutes. Stir. Re-cover. Place in center section of oven and bake for 1½ hours, stirring every 30 minutes. Discard bone; discard bouquet garni after pressing out juices. Taste for salt, adding it if desired.

6. Cut cornbread into wedges, then cut each wedge into 2 equal layers. (Cornbread may be prepared well ahead of time, frozen, and reheated.) Place 3 wedges per serving on warmed individual dinner plates in a circle, with points meeting at center. Spoon portions of stew over cornbread points. Sprinkle with parsley and serve at once.

Yield: **Serves 6**

Note: An electric herb chopper partially chops juniper berries in 1 second.

Serving suggestion: Any green salad completes your meal (pages 173–83).

BRAISED LAMB STEAKS WITH MINT TOMATO SAUCE

For this dish the leanest, meatiest section of the lamb has been braised (cooked with a little stock over low heat after browning). Though it's delicious without adornment, you can raise the dish to a new level of taste with a touch of my Tomato Sauce and some mint for zest.

2 lamb steaks with center bone, ¹/₂ inch thick (about 1 ¹/₂ pounds), each steak cut in half
1 ¹/₂ tablespoons Worcestershire sauce
1 tablespoon Italian olive oil
2 cups Chicken Stock (page 19)
6 sprigs parsley, tied together with cotton thread

2 tablespoons whole dried sage leaves, crushed
1 teaspoon dried mint leaves
2 tablespoons minced shallot
2 teaspoons minced garlic
1 cup Tomato Sauce (page 23)
1 tablespoon minced parsley
¹/₄ teaspoon salt
4 teaspoons dry sherry

1. Damp-wipe meat. Place in wide bowl. Sprinkle all over with Worcestershire sauce. Cover and let stand at room temperature for 45 minutes; or refrigerate for several hours, bringing to room temperature before cooking. Preheat oven to 375 degrees.
2. Heat oil in a well-seasoned iron skillet until quite hot. Add meat. Over medium-high heat, cook on both sides until lightly browned (about 6 minutes). Stir in ³/₄ cup stock. Add parsley bundle, pushing into liquid. Bring to a boil, turning meat several times to coat. Cover tightly and bake in center section of oven until fork-tender, turning and basting 3 times at equal intervals. If liquid evaporates at third turning, add more stock. (Total cooking time will be 60 to 70 minutes, depending upon tenderness of meat.) Finished meat will be a rich brown and almost all liquid will have evaporated.
3. While meat braises, combine sage, mint, shallot, and garlic in medium heavy-bottomed saucepan. Add 1 cup stock. Bring to simmering point. Cover and simmer for 20 minutes. Uncover. Simmer for 2 minutes longer. Strain into a measuring cup, pressing out juices. Measure out ²/₃ cup. Pour back into rinsed-out saucepan.

(Step 3 may be completed up to this point a day ahead and mixture refrigerated.)

4. Pour Tomato Sauce into mixture. Over moderate heat, bring to simmering point. Stir in parsley, salt, and sherry. Simmer, uncovered, over medium heat until sauce is thick and reduced to 1 cup. Remove from heat. Cover and let stand for 5 minutes.

5. Arrange meat on warmed individual serving plates. Ladle each serving with 1 tablespoon sauce. Pour remaining sauce into a gravy-boat and serve along with meat.

Yield: **Serves 4**

CRISPY RACK OF LAMB

Here is the tenderest section of the lamb sealed in a crusty shell of crumbs, herbs, and spices. A far cry from ordinary broiled chops, it's a treat for lamb lovers.

1/2 cup fine bread crumbs (see Note)

1 teaspoon each crushed dried sage leaves and mild curry powder

1/2 teaspoon each cinnamon and freshly grated nutmeg

1/4 teaspoon salt

1 1/2 tablespoons Vegetable Mix (page 18)

1 teaspoon low-sodium soy sauce

1 tablespoon balsamic vinegar

1 tablespoon Italian olive oil

1 tablespoon minced Italian flat parsley

About 1/2 cup fresh orange juice, or unsweetened pineapple juice

1 small rack of lamb (8 rib chops, partially cut through), well trimmed

1. In a small bowl, blend bread crumbs with all seasonings, vegetable mix, soy sauce, vinegar, oil, and parsley, slowly adding enough juice to produce a mealy yet moist mixture. (Combination should hold together when squeezed between 2 fingers.) Reserve remaining juice (about 5 tablespoons).
2. Damp-wipe meat with paper toweling; then rub dry. Spread and press coating over meaty sides of chops, pressing some between each rib. Chill, uncovered, for 30 minutes to set.
3. Preheat oven to 450 degrees. Stand meat in shallow roasting pan (do not use glass). Roast in center section of oven for 15 minutes. Reduce heat to 400 degrees. Dribble with 2 tablespoons juice. Lay sheet of aluminum foil over meat without sealing, and bake for 15 minutes more. Spoon remaining juice over it. Uncover and roast for 10 minutes. Finished meat will be medium-rare with pink interior (overcooking depletes flavor and nutrients). Remove from oven. Cover loosely and let stand for 5 minutes.
4. Cut between chops with sharp serrated knife. Serve on warm individual plates with a portion of crust alongside chops.

Yield: **Serves 4**

Note: The variety of bread used will influence the flavor of the finished dish. I suggest Sourdough French Bread (page 162) or a good-quality commercial rye bread. If you choose the latter, omit salt and include 2 teaspoons of freshly grated Parmesan cheese in Step 1.

Serving suggestions: Couscous with Fruit and Vegetables (page 61); Quinoa Pilaf (page 58).

PORK CHOPS WITH FENNEL

Pork is a savory meat that changes subtly according to the flavors in each new recipe. These lean pork chops are enhanced by Malmsey Madeira and fresh fruit juice. Pork is also reasonably priced and an excellent source of iron and trace minerals.

½ cup raisins
½ to ⅔ cup Malmsey Madeira
4 lean center-cut pork chops (about
 1½ pounds), well trimmed
1 tablespoon Savory Seasoning
 (page 15)
5 teaspoons Italian olive oil
1 tablespoon minced garlic
1 cup ¼-inch pieces fennel (about
 ½ medium bulb)

1 medium red onion, coarsely
 chopped
1 medium sweet green pepper,
 seeded, coarsely chopped
2 tablespoons cider vinegar
¼ cup frozen orange juice
 concentrate
¾ to 1 cup Chicken Stock (page
 19) or water
1 Bouquet Garni (page 16)

1. Place raisins in measuring cup. Add ½ cup Madeira and let soak until plumped up.
2. Damp-wipe chops. Sprinkle and rub with Savory Seasoning. Cover and let stand for 30 minutes. Preheat oven to 325 degrees.
3. Heat 3 teaspoons oil in Dutch oven large enough to hold chops in one layer. Add meat and brown lightly on each side for 4 minutes. Transfer to plate. Heat remaining 2 teaspoons oil. Sauté garlic, fennel, onion, and pepper until softened (about 5 minutes), taking care not to scorch.
4. Pour vinegar around sides of pot. Cook for 1 minute. Combine concentrate with ¾ cup stock or water and add to pot. Drain raisins; strew over mixture. Bring mixture to boil. Drop in Bouquet Garni.
5. Return chops to Dutch oven, turning to coat. Arrange in one layer and reduce heat to simmering. Cover tightly and cook on top of stove for 10 minutes. Then bake until fork-tender (45 to 50 minutes), turning meat and spooning with sauce 3 times at equal intervals. (Cooking time will vary with texture of meat.)
6. Remove from oven. Baste. Re-cover and let stand for 10 minutes before serving. Sauce should be thick. If you prefer a thinner sauce, transfer chops to warm serving plate, then add 2 tablespoons each Madeira and stock to the sauce. Cook over medium-high heat to desired consistency. Spoon over chops and serve at once.

Yield: **Serves 4**

ROAST PORK WITH BABY VEGETABLES

This dish is embellished with colorful baby yellow and green squash and courgettes—as eye-appealing as it is savory. Only 5 minutes to prepare the marinade, only 30 seconds to baste and turn while the meat cooks in the oven, and just a few ticks of the minute hand to compose the sauce (which uses the marinade). It may be one of the easiest dinner party entrées you've ever made!

For the marinade:

1 cup Chicken Stock (page 19)
2 tablespoons frozen pineapple juice
    concentrate
2 teaspoons crushed juniper berries
1 1/2 tablespoons Vegetable Mix
    (page 18)

1 teaspoon each mild curry powder
    and crushed dried sage leaves
1/2 teaspoon each dried thyme
    leaves and cinnamon
4 whole cloves, crushed
1 tablespoon Italian olive oil

For the meat and vegetables:

1 3/4 to 2 pounds boned and
    trimmed center-cut rib of
    pork, rolled to 2 1/2-inch
    diameter
3/4 pound baby vegetables such as
    courgettes and yellow and
    green squash
3/4 cup 1/2-inch cubes white turnip

1 tablespoon sweet
    butter/margarine blend
1/8 teaspoon each nutmeg,
    cinnamon, and salt
1/2 teaspoon prepared Dijon
    mustard, preferably without
    salt

For the sauce:

Reserved marinade
2 teaspoons flavorful honey
1/2 teaspoon prepared Dijon
    mustard, preferably without
    salt

1 tablespoon minced parsley
1/4 teaspoon salt
1 1/2 teaspoons unbleached flour
1 tablespoon Light Choice sour
    cream (optional)

1. In a large nonaluminum bowl, combine 1/2 cup stock with all other marinade ingredients, blending with fork. With sharp-pronged fork, pierce 1/2-inch holes into meat. Place meat in marinade, turning several times to coat. Cover and marinate for 6 hours or overnight in refrigerator, turning twice.

2. Steam vegetables until crisp-tender. Pour into colander and cool under cold running water. Drain and set aside.

3. Preheat oven to 400 degrees. Drain meat, reserving marinade. Place meat on rack in roasting pan. Cover with large sheet of heavy-duty aluminum foil and roast in center section of oven for 20 minutes.

4. Reduce heat to 350 degrees. Roast for 30 minutes longer. Uncover and turn. Baste with 2 tablespoons marinade and pan juices. Re-cover and continue to roast for 40 minutes. Remove from oven and let stand, covered, while sauce is prepared.

5. Pour reserved marinade into heavy-bottomed small saucepan. Bring to simmering point and cook, uncovered, for 7 minutes. Strain through a fine sieve. Pour back into rinsed-out saucepan. Whisk in remaining ½ cup stock, honey, mustard, parsley, and salt. Pour 2 tablespoons sauce into cup. Sprinkle in flour and stir until smooth. Dribble smooth mixture into sauce. Stir and cook until lightly thickened. Keep warm.

6. Thin-slice meat, pouring exuded juices into sauce. Arrange on warm serving platter.

7. To complete cooking vegetables, heat shortening in nonstick skillet until bubbly. Blend in seasonings and mustard. Add vegetables and re-warm over fairly high heat. Place spoonfuls around meat.

8. Whisk sour cream into warm sauce if desired. Ladle over meat, napping vegetables. Serve at once.

Yield: **Serves 4 to 5**

9
SAUCES AND MARINADES

BARBECUE SAUCE

Brushed over uncooked meats and poultry, this fast-cooking sauce seals in flavors and juices and imparts a hearty old-fashioned barbecue taste. Serve it also as a condiment with cooked food.

1 cup unsalted Italian tomato
    puree (see **Note**)
1 tablespoon Savory Seasoning
    (page 15)
¼ teaspoon salt
1½ teaspoons chili con carne
    seasoning
1½ tablespoons firmly packed
    dark brown sugar
2 teaspoons Worcestershire sauce

½ cup cider vinegar
1 teaspoon prepared Dijon mustard
    (preferably without salt)
1 teaspoon dried minced garlic
    (instant garlic)
½ cup minced red onion
1 tablespoon minced fresh coriander
1 tablespoon fresh lemon juice
1 tablespoon Italian olive oil
5 drops Tabasco sauce

1. In a small enameled saucepan, combine all except last 3 ingredients. Bring to simmering point. Cover and cook for 10 minutes.
2. Stir in lemon juice, oil, and Tabasco. Let cool. Store in tightly closed glass jar.

Yield: **About 1¾ cups**

Note: I prefer using canned Italian tomato products because most of them are made from meaty plum tomatoes without added salt or sugar.

QUICK MUSHROOM SAUCE

A zesty sauce for cooked grains, vegetables, grilled meats, fish, and poultry. It also works beautifully as a filling for Pop-Muffins (page 172).

2 tablespoons minced shallot
2 tablespoons cider vinegar
3/4 cup Chicken Stock (page 19)
    or Vegetable Stock (page 20),
    plus 1 tablespoon
1/4 cup Malmsey Madeira
4 medium snow-white fresh
    mushrooms, trimmed,
    damp-wiped, finely chopped

(about 1 cup)
1/4 teaspoon each ground ginger
    and mild curry powder
1 tablespoon minced parsley or
    fresh coriander
1/8 to 1/4 teaspoon salt
2 teaspoons cornstarch or
    arrowroot
2 tablespoons milk

1. Combine shallot and vinegar in small heavy-bottomed saucepan. Bring to simmering point. Cook, uncovered, until all liquid evaporates.
2. Stir in 3/4 cup stock, wine, mushrooms, spices, and parsley or coriander. Bring to a boil. Reduce heat to simmering. Cover and simmer for 12 minutes. Stir in 1/8 teaspoon salt.
3. In a cup, combine cornstarch with remaining 1 tablespoon stock, stirring until smooth. While stirring, dribble mixture into sauce. Cook for 2 minutes. Add milk; simmer for 2 minutes, stirring continually. Taste for salt, adding remaining 1/8 teaspoon if desired. Serve at once.

Yield: **About 1 cup**

DUXELLE SAUCE

Duxelles are minced mushrooms cooked with Madeira. A touch of cayenne, sherry, and stock makes an elegant mushroom sauce that flatters every food it touches.

2 tablespoons minced shallot
2 tablespoons dry sherry or cider vinegar
1 cup Chicken Stock (page 19) or Vegetable Stock (page 20)
1/4 cup Madeira Duxelles (page 59)

1 tablespoon minced parsley
Up to 1/4 teaspoon salt
Cayenne pepper
2 teaspoons arrowroot or cornstarch, dissolved in 1 tablespoon water

1. In a small heavy-bottomed saucepan, combine shallot and sherry or vinegar. Cook, uncovered, over low heat until all liquid evaporates.
2. Stir in stock. Bring to a boil. Reduce heat to simmering. Add duxelles, parsley, and salt. Simmer, uncovered, for 5 minutes. Sprinkle in cayenne pepper to taste.
3. Drizzle in thickening mixture. Cook for 2 minutes over moderate heat. Serve at once in warmed gravy boat along with food.

Yield: **About 1 cup**

LUMP CRABMEAT SAUCE WITH FENNEL

A creamy, rich-tasting sauce with bits of fresh crabmeat. It's perfect over just-toasted bread or hot rice, or for spooning around broiled fish or Scrod Fish Cakes (page 119).

½ pound fresh lump crabmeat,
    picked over
1 tablespoon fresh lemon juice
3 ripe plum tomatoes
2 teaspoons fennel seed, crushed
2½ tablespoons sweet
    butter/margarine blend
2 tablespoons minced shallot
2 teaspoons mild curry powder
½ teaspoon freshly grated nutmeg

3 tablespoons unbleached flour
¾ cups Fish Stock (page 21)
2 tablespoons dry sherry
⅛ teaspoon cayenne pepper
¼ cup milk
3 tablespoons light cream
2 tablespoons minced parsley
⅛ to ¼ teaspoon salt
Freshly ground white or black
    pepper to taste

1. Place crabmeat in small bowl. Separate lumps without flaking. Sprinkle with lemon juice, stirring to coat. Set aside.
2. Drop tomatoes into a saucepan of boiling water. Cook for 2 minutes. When cool enough to handle, remove skin. Core and squeeze out seeds; cut up. Place in food blender with fennel and purée. Measure out ½ cup, reserving balance for another recipe.
3. Heat shortening in a medium heavy-bottomed saucepan. Over moderate heat, sauté shallots for 1 minute. Sprinkle in spices. Stir and continue to sauté until shallots are wilted but not brown. Combine flour with mixture and cook for 1 minute.
4. Gradually add stock, stirring and cooking until mixture thickens. Then stir in puréed tomatoes, sherry, and cayenne pepper. While stirring, dribble in milk and cream; add parsley and ⅛ teaspoon salt. Bring to simmering point. Simmer, uncovered, for 2 minutes. Fold in crabmeat and cook only until heated through. Add pepper. Taste for salt, adding remaining ⅛ teaspoon if desired. Serve at once.

Yield: **2 cups**

HOT CRANBERRY GRAVY

Unlike typical poultry dressings, this gravy is prepared *without* poultry. So, it's equally good over roast meats, grains, or potatoes.

¾ cup Chicken Stock (page 19)
    or Vegetable Stock (page 20)
⅓ cup fresh cranberries, rinsed
    and drained
1 tablespoon frozen orange juice
    concentrate
1 tablespoon sugar
2 teaspoons each Italian olive oil

and sweet butter/margarine
    blend
¼ teaspoon mild curry powder
½ teaspoon cinnamon
⅛ to ¼ teaspoon salt
4½ teaspoons unbleached flour
¼ to ½ cup combined whole and
    low-fat milk

1. In a small heavy-bottomed saucepan, combine stock, cranberries, concentrate, and sugar. Bring to a boil. Reduce heat to simmering. Cover partially and simmer for 10 minutes. Pour into a bowl; set aside. Rinse out saucepan.
2. Combine shortening and oil in saucepan. Heat to bubbling. Sprinkle in spices and salt. Stir and cook for 1 minute. Add flour. Over moderate heat, cook and stir for 1 minute longer. Pour cranberry mixture into gravy gradually. Bring to simmering point. Cook, uncovered, for 2 minutes.
3. While stirring continually, pour in milk a little at a time, until smooth and thickened. Use remaining milk, if necessary, to thin to desired consistency.

Yield: **About 1 cup; recipe may be doubled**

Note: Recipe may be prepared through Step 1 several hours or a day ahead and completed just before serving.

FRESH HORSERADISH SAUCE

This lusty "cream" sauce derives most of its flavor from fresh horseradish root. It complements braised or roasted meats and poultry, and its naturally biting flavor is a fine foil for steamed or broiled fish. Try the variation, too; puréed beets tame down the sauce's sharp edge and transform its color to hot-pink.

About 5 ounces fresh horseradish, peeled
2 tablespoons white wine vinegar
½ cup low-fat buttermilk, preferably unsalted

¼ cup Light Choice sour cream
¼ teaspoon salt
½ teaspoon freshly ground black pepper

1. Fit food processor with grating blade. Cut horseradish into uniform pieces and grate. Re-fit workbowl with steel blade. Process until horseradish is chopped to the size of pinheads. Scrape into a bowl.
2. Add vinegar, stirring to blend. Then combine with remaining ingredients. Transfer to a jar. Cover and let stand at room temperature for one hour before serving. Store unused sauce in refrigerator for up to 5 days.

Yield: **1½ cups**

Variation: Prepare basic recipe. Purée a drained unsalted 8-ounce can of sliced beets in food blender or processor, using 2 tablespoons of the canned juices. Measure out ⅓ cup of the puree and add to the sauce. Increase vinegar measurement to 3 tablespoons and stir in 6 finely crushed cloves. Let stand for 1 hour before serving.

RAISIN SAUCE

When you want a touch of sweet creaminess—without cream—over meat, fish, poultry, and grains. I use this sauce with Veal Florentine (page 130).

1/4 cup raisins
1/4 cup finely minced shallots
2 cups Chicken Stock (page 19) or
    Vegetable Stock (page 20)
1 1/2 tablespoons balsamic vinegar
1 tablespoon minced parsley
1/8 teaspoon each freshly grated
    nutmeg and salt

1 teaspoon dried tarragon leaves,
    crumbled
1 tablespoon dry sherry
1 teaspoon sweet butter/margarine
    blend
2 teaspoons cornstarch
2 tablespoons milk or light cream

1. In a small heavy-bottomed saucepan, combine raisins, shallots, 1 1/4 cups stock, vinegar, and parsley. Bring to simmering point. Simmer, uncovered, until reduced to 3/4 cup. Strain, pressing out juices. Discard solids. Pour sauce back into saucepan.
2. Add remaining 3/4 cup stock, seasonings, and sherry. Simmer gently for 5 minutes. Stir in shortening.
3. Measure cornstarch into a cup. Add milk slowly and stir until very smooth. Gradually dribble half into the hot sauce, stirring until mixture begins to thicken slightly. Add enough of the remaining mixture to thicken sauce to desired texture.

Yield: **About 1 cup**

JUNIPER BERRY MARINADE

Imparts a velvety, distinctively seasoned coating to roast or clay-pot chicken or meat. Delicious, too, brushed over meat or skinned chicken before broiling.

1 tablespoon balsamic vinegar
2 tablespoons frozen pineapple juice
    concentrate
1 teaspoon each dry mustard and
    mild curry powder
1/4 teaspoon salt
2 tablespoons fresh lime juice

1 tablespoon Vegetable Mix (page
    18)
2 tablespoons crushed juniper
    berries
1/4 cup low-fat buttermilk,
    preferably without salt

1. In a small bowl, whisk vinegar and concentrate until well blended. Then whisk in seasonings, salt, and lime juice.
2. Stir in Vegetable Mix, juniper berries, and buttermilk. Let stand for 5 minutes; stir again before using.

Yield: **About 3/4 cup (enough to marinate a 3 1/2-pound chicken or a boned roast)**

Note: If salted buttermilk is used, eliminate salt from recipe.

WINE MARINADE

A delicious marinade for lamb, beef, or pork. Try it, too, as a basting liquid for broilings.

1/4 cup red wine
2 teaspoons balsamic vinegar
2 teaspoons low-sodium soy sauce
1 tablespoon Savory Seasoning
    (page 15)

1/2 teaspoon minced fresh ginger
1 teaspoon minced garlic
2 tablespoons minced shallot
1 tablespoon minced parsley
Pinch salt

1. In a small bowl, whisk together wine, vinegar, soy sauce, and seasoning.
2. Stir in remaining ingredients. Let stand for 15 minutes. Stir again before using.

Yield: **About 1/2 cup (enough to marinate a 3 1/2-pound boned roast or 4 chops)**

10
BREADS AND MUFFINS

OAT CRACKERS

Have your fiber and enjoy it too! Pure oatmeal and oat bran, moistened with apple juice and water, are flavored with cinnamon and sesame seed. Serve these crackers with soups and salads, or alone as a satisfying snack. They go well with Spicy Peanut Spread, too (page 44).

1 cup plus 2 tablespoons oat bran
1 1/2 cups plus 2 tablespoons rolled oats
2 tablespoons unhulled sesame seeds (available in health-food stores)

1/2 teaspoon cinnamon
1/4 teaspoon salt (optional)
1/2 cup cold apple juice
1/4 cup cold water
1 tablespoon peanut oil

1. Preheat oven to 275 degrees. In a large bowl, combine 1 cup oat bran, 1 1/2 cups rolled oats, sesame seeds, and seasonings. Combine juice with water. Pour over mixture, stirring until dough begins to congeal. Sprinkle with oil. Combine with hands, compressing until dough forms a fairly stable mass.
2. Combine remaining 2 tablespoons each bran and rolled oats in a cup. Sprinkle board with half the mixture. Lay dough on top of mix and, using mild pressure, press with heel of hands to a rectangular shape. With a rolling pin, roll out to an 8 × 12-inch rectangle. (Ideally, it should be rolled to 1/4-inch thickness.) Fill cracks with some of remaining oat bran/rolled oats mix as you roll. Cut away ragged edges.
3. Cut crosswise into long 1 1/2-inch strips. With a spatula, scoop up each strip and place on ungreased cookie sheet. Using a blunt knife, make partial cuts into dough every 1 1/2 to 2 inches. Bake for 30 minutes. Turn each strip carefully. Bake for 20 minutes—5 minutes longer for those sections of crackers that are thicker than 1/4 inch.
4. Place strips on rack. Break through indentations. Let cool completely before serving. Store in tightly closed tin.

Yield: **About 3 dozen crackers**

Note: These crackers will have a pleasing homemade look, and they don't contain bad fats and excess salt.

MASTERPIECE BREAD (AND SWEET BUNS)

Here's your chance to become an instant master baker, even if you've never baked before. All you need is this foolproof combination of ingredients and your food processor. The masterpiece you'll bake will be a delicate, cake-textured, sweet-tasting loaf. Try the Sweet Buns too.

3 tablespoons flavorful honey
1/4 cup warm water (105 to 115 degrees)
About 2 1/4 cups unbleached flour
1 package dry yeast
3/4 cup fresh orange juice
2 tablespoons walnut or peanut oil
1/2 cup stone-ground whole wheat flour
1/4 cup oat bran

2 tablespoons regular wheat germ
3/4 teaspoon salt
1 teaspoon non-aluminum baking powder
2 tablespoons nonfat dry milk solids
1/4 teaspoon each allspice and freshly grated nutmeg
1 tablespoon milk

1. In a tall water glass, combine and blend with fork 1 tablespoon honey, water, 2 tablespoons unbleached flour, and yeast. Let stand until mixture foams and rises to top of glass (7 to 10 minutes).
2. In a small saucepan, combine and heat juice, remaining 2 tablespoons honey, and oil until moderately warm. Set aside.
3. In workbowl of food processor fitted with a steel blade, place 1 3/4 cups unbleached flour, whole wheat flour, oat bran, wheat germ, salt, baking powder, milk solids, and spices. Process in 4 on/off turns. With machine running, pour risen yeast mixture through feed tube, scraping out glass. Process for 10 seconds. Then pour juice mixture through feed tube and process until dough forms into a ball and rotates around bowl 10 times. Remove cover of workbowl; sprinkle with 3 tablespoons flour. Re-cover and process until ball rotates around bowl 25 times. Stop machine.
4. Transfer dough to very lightly floured board. Knead briefly by hand, folding dough over while making quarter turns, pushing each time with heel of hand. If still sticky, sprinkle with 1 teaspoon of flour at a time while kneading until moist to the touch but not sticky. Shape into a ball.
5. Lightly oil a medium, fairly straight-sided warmed bowl. Drop ball

in, turning to coat. Cover tightly with plastic wrap. Let rise at room temperature (70 to 80 degrees) until doubled (about 1½ hours). Punch down. Knead briefly on board. Shape into a ball. Cover and let rest for 5 minutes.

6. Flatten dough into a rectangle wide enough to fit an 8-inch loaf pan. Roll up tightly lengthwise, pinching seam and ends. Lightly grease pan with sweet butter/margarine blend. Place loaf, seam down, in pan. Cover with lightly greased sheet of wax paper. Let rise until doubled (1¼ to 1½ hours). Preheat oven to 375 degrees.

7. Bake in center section of oven for 15 minutes. Reduce heat to 350 degrees. Cover loaf loosely with aluminum foil. Bake for 20 minutes. Loosen around sides of pan with blunt knife and carefully remove bread. If bottom of loaf produces a hollow sound when tapped with knuckles, bread is done. If not, place loaf directly onto oven rack and bake 5 minutes more. Remove from oven and place on rack. Brush tops and sides with milk. Let cool completely if thin slices are desired, or serve warm, cut into thick slices.

Yield: **1 loaf**

Variation: Sweet Buns (1 dozen)

After completing recipe through Step 5, roll dough to an 11 × 14-inch rectangle on an unfloured surface. Spread with 2 teaspoons soft sweet butter/margarine blend. In a cup, combine ¼ cup each raisins and coarsely chopped walnuts, 2 teaspoons cinnamon, ½ teaspoon ground cardamom, and 2 tablespoons date powder or dark brown sugar. Sprinkle evenly over dough, leaving a ½-inch border. Roll up tightly, pinching seam to seal.

With a sharp serrated knife, cut into twelve ½-inch slices (dough pulls back to smaller dimension after rolling). Place on butter/margarine–greased 13 × 9 × 2-inch cookie tin, spacing evenly. Cover with lightly oiled sheet of wax paper. Let rise in warm place until doubled.

Bake in preheated 375-degree oven until golden (about 15 minutes). Place pan on rack. Brush immediately with a mixture of 2 tablespoons each flavorful honey and fresh orange juice. Transfer buns to rack and cool to warm.

BUTTERMILK WHOLE WHEAT BREAD

Spongy, molasses- and spice-sweetened, and given a shade of tartness with buttermilk, these loaves bear no resemblance to commercial whole wheat bread.

1 teaspoon plus 1 tablespoon flavorful honey
1/3 cup warm water (105 to 115 degrees)
About 1 3/4 cups unbleached flour
1 package dry yeast
1 cup unsalted low-fat buttermilk
2 tablespoons unsulphured molasses
2 tablespoons sweet

butter/margarine blend
1 1/2 cups stone-ground whole wheat flour
1 tablespoon nonfat dry milk solids
1/2 teaspoon non-aluminum baking powder
1/4 teaspoon each cinnamon and ground cardamom
1/2 teaspoon salt

1. In a tall water glass, combine and blend with fork 1 teaspoon honey, water, 2 tablespoons flour, and yeast. Let stand until mixture foams and rises to top of glass (7 to 10 minutes).
2. In a small saucepan, over low heat, combine and warm buttermilk, molasses, remaining tablespoon honey, and shortening, taking care not to overheat. Set aside.
3. In workbowl of food processor fitted with a steel blade, place 1 1/2 cups unbleached flour, whole wheat flour, milk solids, baking powder, spices, and salt. Process in 4 on/off turns. With machine running, pour risen yeast mixture through feed tube, scraping out glass. Process for 10 seconds. Then pour through warm buttermilk mixture and process until ball forms and rotates around the bowl 10 times. Remove cover of workbowl; sprinkle with remaining 2 tablespoons flour. Re-cover and process until ball rotates around bowl 25 times.
4. Transfer to board and knead briefly by hand. Dough should not be sticky. If it is, sprinkle board with 1 to 2 teaspoons flour and knead by hand, folding dough over while making quarter turns, pushing each time with heel of hand. Shape into a ball.
5. Lightly oil a medium, fairly straight-sided warmed bowl. Drop ball in, turning to coat. Cover tightly with plastic wrap. Let rise at room temperature (70 to 80 degrees) until doubled (1 1/4 to 1 1/2 hours). Punch down. Knead briefly. Shape into a ball. Cover and let rest for 5 minutes.

6. Flatten dough into a rectangle wide enough to fit an 8- or 9-inch loaf pan. Roll up tightly lengthwise, pinching seam and ends. Grease pan lightly with sweet butter/margarine blend. Place loaf, seam down, in pan. Cover with a sheet of lightly greased wax paper. Let rise until doubled (1 ¼ to 1 ½ hours). Preheat oven to 375 degrees. **7.** Bake in center section of oven for 15 minutes. Reduce heat to 350 degrees. Cover loosely with a sheet of aluminum foil. Bake for 25 minutes. Place pan on rack for 3 minutes. Loosen around sides of pan with blunt knife and remove bread carefully. If bottom of loaf produces a hollow sound when tapped with knuckles, bread is done. If not, place loaf directly onto oven rack and bake 5 minutes more. Place on rack. Let cool completely before slicing.

Yield: **1 loaf**

ANADAMA OATMEAL BREAD

This is my version of the classic bread created by the unappreciated wife of a whaling captain whose ship is now on permanent exhibit on the San Francisco waterfront. He referred to her as "Anna, damn her," from which the bread takes its name. My modern loaves, nutrition-boosted by oatmeal, are proud and plump and sweet, just as I imagine Anna must have been. Textured like cake, this bread is the base for a superlative French Toast (page 211). It also makes fine bread crumbs.

2 1/2 cups water
1/2 teaspoon sugar
2 packages dry yeast
3 tablespoons frozen apple juice
    concentrate
1/3 cup each stone-ground yellow
    cornmeal and rolled oats
1 teaspoon salt
1/4 cup unsulphured molasses
1 tablespoon each Italian olive oil

and sweet butter/margarine
    blend
5 1/2 to 6 cups unbleached flour
1/2 teaspoon each ground coriander
    and cinnamon
1/2 teaspoon non-aluminum baking
    powder
1 teaspoon sweet butter/margarine
    blend, melted (optional)

1. In a medium-size heavy-bottomed saucepan, heat water to warm (105 to 115 degrees). Pour 1/4 cup water into large bowl of mixing machine. Sprinkle with sugar, stirring to dissolve. Add yeast, beating with fork to blend. Let stand for 8 minutes to proof (mixture should puff up).
2. Stir concentrate into remaining water in saucepan. Bring to a boil. Sprinkle in cornmeal (as you would for making cream of wheat), and whisk vigorously to prevent lumps from forming. Stir in rolled oats, salt, molasses, oil, and shortening. Boil for 1 minute. Remove from heat and let cool to tepid, stirring often to hasten cooling (mixture will be thick). Pour into yeast mixture and blend with wooden spoon.
3. Stir in 2 cups flour, spices, and baking powder. Using paddle attachment of mixing machine, beat on medium speed for 2 minutes. Remove bowl from base of mixing machine and using wooden spoon, beat in 3 cups unbleached flour, 1/2 cup at a time, beating well after each addition. When dough becomes too difficult to handle with spoon, set bowl on base of mixing machine and, using dough hook,

knead at low setting, adding flour a little at a time until dough cleans sides of bowl. Continue kneading for 5 minutes. (If you're kneading by hand, when dough becomes too difficult to handle with wooden spoon, scoop up and turn onto lightly floured board and knead, adding up to 4 cups remaining flour, ½ cup at a time, to make a smooth elastic dough. Bulk will diminish as kneading continues. Whether you're using a dough hook or kneading by hand, add only enough flour to make a dough that's smooth and elastic and no longer sticky.)

4. Shape dough into a ball. Drop into a lightly oiled, fairly straight-sided large mixing bowl, turning to coat. Cover tightly with plastic wrap. Let stand at room temperature (70 to 80 degrees) until more than double in bulk (about 1½ hours).

5. Punch down. Turn onto a lightly floured board and knead briefly, squeezing out bubbles. Cut into two pieces and shape into balls. Cover loosely with wax paper and let rest for 5 minutes. With hands, shape each ball into a 7 × 10-inch rectangle. Roll up tightly, pinching seams and tucking in ends. Place in 2 lightly greased 8- or 9-inch loaf pans. Lightly oil a large sheet of wax paper. Cover bread, loosely tucking in ends. Let rise at room temperature until well above sides of pans (about 1¼ hours). Preheat oven to 400 degrees.

6. Place loaves in center section of oven. Bake for 10 minutes. Reduce heat to 350 degrees and continue baking for 30 minutes longer, checking after 15 minutes to see if tops are browning too rapidly. If so, cover loosely with a sheet of aluminum foil. Remove bread from pans. Tap bottom of loaves. A hollow sound indicates that bread is fully baked. If not, place loaves directly on rack in oven and bake for 5 minutes more. Brush immediately with shortening, if desired. Cool completely on rack. Turn loaves on their sides and slice with a sharp serrated knife, taking care not to exert too much pressure.

Yield: **2 large plump loaves**

SOURDOUGH FRENCH BREAD

This is a sourdough bread—which means an ever-so-slightly-tart loaf—the kind preferred by some of the most serious bread lovers in the world, San Franciscans.

For the starter:

2 packages dry yeast
1/2 teaspoon sugar
2 cups warm water (105 to 115
    degrees)

2 cups unbleached flour
1/2 cup rye flour
1/4 cup nonfat dry milk solids

For the dough:

1 cup unsweetened apple juice
1/2 cup water
1 teaspoon salt
1/2 cup rye flour
3 tablespoons finely crushed
    coriander seeds

6 to 6 3/4 cups unbleached flour
1/3 cup freshly grated Parmesan
    cheese
1 egg white, mixed with 1
    tablespoon water
Unhulled sesame seeds

1. Two days before baking, sprinkle yeast and sugar into a large mixing bowl. Add water and stir with a fork to blend. Add flours and milk solids. Blend well with wooden spoon. Cover tightly with plastic wrap, and let stand until baking day, stirring down after 24 hours and then re-covering tightly. Mixture will bubble up and then settle down and will give off a slightly sour but not unpleasant aroma.
2. To prepare dough, stir starter. Combine juice, water, and salt in a saucepan and heat to 105 to 115 degrees. Pour over the starter and beat with wooden spoon until blended.
3. Add rye flour and coriander seeds and stir. Stir in 6 cups unbleached flour, 1/2 cup at a time, beating well after each addition, adding Parmesan cheese after 3 cups flour have been incorporated. When dough becomes too difficult to handle with wooden spoon, set bowl on base of mixing machine and, using dough hook, knead at low setting, scraping down sides of bowl periodically and adding flour, 1/2 cup at a time, until dough cleans sides of bowl. Continue kneading for 5 minutes. (If you're kneading by hand, when dough becomes too difficult to handle with a wooden spoon, scoop it up and turn it onto

a lightly floured board and knead, adding up to a total of 6 cups flour, ½ cup at a time, to make a smooth elastic dough. Bulk will diminish as kneading continues. Whether you're using a dough hook or kneading by hand, add only enough flour to make a dough that's still slightly sticky but works into a pliant loose ball.)

4. Drop the ball into an ungreased, fairly straight-sided bowl. Cover with a very lightly oiled plastic wrap. Let stand at room temperature (70 to 80 degrees) until more than double in bulk. Punch down and knead briefly in bowl, sprinkling with 1 tablespoon flour if dough remains very sticky. Re-cover and let rise again until doubled.

5. Punch down. Scrape dough out of bowl onto lightly floured board and knead for a few turns. For easier kneading, cut dough in half, and knead each piece separately, squeezing out air bubbles (you'll hear them pop). Cut each piece in half and shape into balls. Cover loosely with wax paper and let rest for 5 minutes. With hands, shape each ball into a 5 × 10-inch rectangle. Fold over lengthwise, pinching seam. Roll back and forth until each loaf is rounded and stretched to 14 inches long.

6. Grease four 14-inch French bread pans with small amount of sweet butter/margarine blend. Lay loaves in pan. With sharp serrated knife, slash each loaf diagonally in four places. Brush with egg wash. Lightly oil long sheets of wax paper to cover pans, loosely tucking in ends. Let rise at room temperature until double in bulk (about 50 minutes). Preheat oven to 450 degrees. Half-fill a roasting pan with boiling water and slide onto the bottom of oven. When bread is fully risen, gently brush again with egg wash and sprinkle with sesame seeds.

7. Bake loaves for 15 minutes. Shift position of pans so that bread bakes evenly. Reduce oven heat to 375 degrees and bake until browned (25 to 30 minutes). Remove pans and tap bottom of loaves. A hollow sound indicates that bread is done. If not, place bread directly onto oven rack and bake for a few minutes longer. Cool completely on rack before slicing.

Yield: **4 loaves**

Notes:

1. Three rises produces a fine-textured crumb. The second rise may be eliminated if you prefer a coarse-textured crumb.

2. Because no shortening is used, bread will remain fresh for only one day. It does, however, freeze well. Wrap in plastic film and then in aluminum foil. To reheat, remove plastic, rewrap in foil, and bake in preheated 375-degree oven for 15 minutes. Remove from foil and let cool for 2 to 3 minutes before slicing.

SPICED BANANA BREAD

A perennial favorite that could, with the addition of a glass of skim milk and fruit, constitute your first meal of the day.

3 tablespoons sweet
  butter/margarine blend
1 tablespoon peanut oil
1/4 cup plus 1 teaspoon firmly
  packed light or dark brown
  sugar
2 tablespoons frozen orange or
  pineapple juice concentrate
2 medium ripe bananas, sliced
3 eggs, separated (use 2 yolks and
  3 whites)
1 teaspoon pure vanilla extract

2 1/4 cups unbleached flour
2 1/2 teaspoons non-aluminum
  baking powder
1/2 teaspoon each ground ginger
  and cinnamon
1/4 cup each plain low-fat yogurt
  and milk
1/8 teaspoon cream of tartar
1/2 teaspoon each cinnamon and
  freshly grated nutmeg
1/4 cup coarsely chopped walnuts

1. Preheat oven to 350 degrees. In large bowl of mixing machine, combine shortening, oil, and sugar. Beat on medium speed until well blended. Add concentrate and beat for 30 seconds. Then add bananas, beating until absorbed into mixture. Drop yolks into shortening mix and whites into another mixing machine bowl. Combine vanilla with shortening mix.
2. Sift flour, baking powder, and spices into a bowl. Set aside.
3. Combine yogurt and milk. While beating on moderate speed, add to batter alternately with dry ingredients.
4. Beat egg whites on moderate speed until foamy. Sprinkle in cream of tartar. Beat on highest speed until firm but not dry peaks form. With wooden spoon, stir one-third into batter; fold in balance.
5. Lightly grease a 9-inch loose-bottomed tube pan with shortening. Spoon batter into pan. In a cup, combine remaining 1 teaspoon sugar with spices and walnuts. Sprinkle over cake. With blunt knife, fold mix into batter in 5 or 6 places (do not mix), smoothing out top. Bake for 45 to 50 minutes. Test for doneness: A toothpick inserted into center should come out clean. Place pan on rack and let cool for 5 minutes. Loosen around sides of pan. Lift out tube section and cool on rack. Let bread completely cool before removing from pan.

Yield: **1 loaf**

BREAKFAST CORNBREAD

This is a light, smooth, delicately flavored cornbread—utterly different from its traditional butter-laden, sugar-heavy counterpart. That's because I've prepared it with low-fat buttermilk, and sweetened it with freshly grated nutmeg and apple juice concentrate.

1 teaspoon sweet butter/margarine
  blend
2 cups yellow cornmeal
1 cup unbleached flour
2 1/2 teaspoons non-aluminum
  baking powder
1 teaspoon baking soda
1/4 teaspoon salt

1/2 teaspoon freshly grated nutmeg
2 large eggs
1 tablespoon frozen apple juice
  concentrate
4 teaspoons sweet butter/margarine
  blend, melted
2 1/2 to 2 2/3 cups low-fat
  buttermilk, preferably unsalted

1. Preheat oven to 400 degrees. Grease an 8- or 9-inch-square baking pan with shortening. Place pan in hot oven for 4 minutes.
2. Sift cornmeal, flour, baking powder, baking soda, salt, and spices into a large bowl. In another bowl, combine and whisk eggs, concentrate, and 3 teaspoons melted butter. Stir in 2 1/2 cups milk.
3. Combine liquid mixture with dry ingredients, stirring with wooden spoon until batter is moist, adding remaining milk, if necessary, to make a thick yet pourable batter.
4. Pour batter into prepared hot pan, spreading well into corners. Place in center section of oven and bake for 25 minutes. Finished bread should be lightly browned and start to pull away from sides of pan. Brush top with remaining 1 teaspoon butter. Stand pan on rack for 5 minutes. Cut into 16 squares. Serve warm.

Yield: **Serves 8**

Variation: For a subtle change in taste, substitute frozen pineapple or orange juice concentrate for apple juice concentrate.

Note: This cornbread and Dinner Cornbread (page 166) freeze exceptionally well. Wrap squares in foil, freeze, and reheat (in foil) in a preheated 400-degree oven for about 15 minutes.

DINNER CORNBREAD

For a delectable accompaniment to main courses of meat or poultry, I've added sautéed peppers, shallot, and Savory Seasoning to the traditional recipe. It's a lighter-than-usual cornbread, because I've folded beaten egg whites into the batter. Makes a fine stuffing, too (see recipe for Stuffed Cornish Hens, page 80).

2 tablespoons Italian olive oil
3 tablespoons each coarsely chopped sweet red pepper and shallot
1 1/2 teaspoons Savory Seasoning (page 15)
1 1/2 cups stone-ground yellow cornmeal
1 1/2 cups unbleached flour
3 teaspoons non-aluminum baking powder

1/2 teaspoon baking soda
2 eggs, separated
1/2 cup each skim milk and whole milk (or all low-fat milk, 1% milk fat)
2 teaspoons sweet butter/margarine blend, melted
3 tablespoons freshly grated Parmesan cheese

1. Preheat oven to 400 degrees. Heat oil in small nonstick skillet. Add pepper and shallot; sprinkle with Savory Seasoning. Sauté over medium heat until wilted and mixture begins to brown. Set aside.
2. Sift cornmeal, flour, baking powder, and baking soda into a large bowl. In another bowl, combine egg yolks and milk, blending with fork. Stir in melted shortening.
3. Add egg mixture and sautéed vegetables to dry ingredients. Sprinkle in Parmesan cheese. Combine with wooden spoon until batter is moist. Mixture will be fairly thick.
4. Beat egg whites until firm but not dry peaks form. Stir one-third into batter; fold in remainder.
5. Grease an 8- or 9-inch square baking pan lightly with butter/margarine blend. Spread batter across pan and well into corners. Place in center section of preheated oven and bake for 25 minutes. Stand on rack and let cool for 5 minutes. Cut into 16 squares. Serve warm.

Yield: **Serves 8**

BREAKFAST CAKE BREAD

This flavorsome hybrid is more cake than bread and more bread than cake—depending on your taste. A combination of poppy seeds, yogurt, spices, and two flours, it's perfect for breakfast.

1 1/2 cups unbleached flour
1/2 cup stone-ground whole wheat flour
1/2 teaspoon each cinnamon and ground coriander
2 teaspoons non-aluminum baking powder
1/2 teaspoon baking soda
1 cup plain low-fat yogurt, room temperature
1/4 cup milk (skim or regular)
3 tablespoons poppy seeds

3 tablespoons sweet butter/margarine blend, plus 1 teaspoon
2 tablespoons peanut oil
1/4 cup each loosely packed light brown sugar and granulated sugar
1 tablespoon frozen orange juice concentrate
3 eggs (use 1 yolk and 3 whites)
1 tablespoon grated orange rind
Pinch cream of tartar

1. Preheat oven to 350 degrees. Sift first 5 listed ingredients into a bowl. Set aside.
2. Combine yogurt and milk in a small heavy-bottomed saucepan. Heat over lowest stove setting until warm (do not boil). Stir in poppy seeds. Set aside.
3. Put shortening, oil, sugar, and date powder in large bowl of mixing machine. Beat on highest speed until well blended. Add concentrate and beat for 30 seconds. Reduce speed. Separate eggs, dropping 1 yolk into mixture and 3 whites into another mixing machine bowl. Beat in dry ingredients alternately with warmed yogurt mix. Sprinkle in orange rind and blend.
4. Beat egg whites until foamy. Add cream of tartar. Increase speed to highest setting and beat until firm but not dry peaks form. Fold into batter.
5. Grease a 9-inch loose-bottomed tube pan lightly. Spread batter into pan. Bake in center section of preheated oven for 45 to 50 minutes. Test for doneness: A toothpick inserted into center should come out clean. Place pan on rack and let cool for 5 minutes. With a blunt knife, loosen around sides. Lift out tube section and place on rack. When completely cool, remove bread from pan. Plastic-wrap and let flavors develop overnight.

Yield: 10 to 12 servings

MUFFINS

A quartet of breakfast treats. All-American favorites, probably because of their wide range of flavors and textures, muffins are the easiest to prepare of all baked products. Here are my Apple-Bran Muffins, Buckwheat Muffins, sweet and savory Banana-Oat Muffins.

Plus—Pop-Muffins. These have the soft, hollow interior of popovers and the sturdy crust of muffins. To ensure their success every time, pay keen attention to oven heat. Most important: No peeking until they're completely baked!

APPLE-BRAN MUFFINS

1 ³/₄ cups unbleached flour
2 ¹/₂ teaspoons non-aluminum
  baking powder
¹/₂ teaspoon each cinnamon and
  ground cardamom
2 tablespoons nonfat dry milk
  solids
¹/₂ cup oat bran
2 tablespoons each sugar and
  flavorful honey

1 large egg
1 cup fresh orange juice
¹/₄ cup peanut oil
¹/₂ teaspoon pure vanilla extract
2 tablespoons Light Choice sour
  cream or plain low-fat yogurt
2 crisp medium apples, such as
  Washington State, peeled,
  cored, cut into ¹/₂-inch cubes

1. Preheat oven to 375 degrees. Sift flour, baking powder, and spices into a large bowl. Stir in milk solids, oat bran, and sugar.
2. In a small bowl, with fork, beat honey lightly with egg. Stir in juice and oil. Make a well in the center of the dry mix. Add liquids and stir only until dry mix is moistened. In a cup, combine extract with sour cream or yogurt and add to batter. Fold in apples.
3. Grease 12 muffin cups lightly with sweet butter/margarine blend. Fill each cup with equal amounts of batter (yield will be affected by volume of apples). Bake until muffins are lightly brown and begin to pull away from sides of cups (20 to 23 minutes).
4. Place pan on rack to cool for 5 minutes. With a blunt knife, loosen each muffin around sides. Lift out of cups gently (they're fragile) and place on rack. Serve warm.

Yield: **12 muffins**

Variation: Crisp pears, such as Bosc, may be substituted for apples; add ¹/₄ teaspoon freshly grated nutmeg to recipe.

Notes for all muffin recipes:

1. Have all ingredients at room temperature.
2. Use a large wooden spoon or wide flexible spatula to combine ingredients.
3. Stir or fold in ingredients, rather than beating them.
4. Preheat oven for at least 10 minutes before baking.
5. Position oven rack in center of stove; place pan in center of rack to ensure even baking.
6. Fill muffin cups three-quarters full for yield of one dozen 3-inch muffins; fill cups to the top for 9 large, over-the-brim muffins, greasing surface areas between depressions of pan for easy removal without breaking.
7. For crunchy exteriors, and more pointed flavors, grease cups lightly with butter/margarine blend rather than filling with paper liners.
8. For extra sweetness and gloss, brush finished muffins with a mixture of 1 tablespoon flavorful honey dissolved in 1 tablespoon warm fruit juice.
9. Freeze muffins wrapped in foil, and reheat in foil in a preheated 400-degree oven for about 15 minutes.

BUCKWHEAT MUFFINS

1 1/4 cups unbleached flour
1/2 cup buckwheat flour (see
  Notes)
1/4 cup stone-ground whole wheat
  flour
2 tablespoons cornstarch
2 teaspoons non-aluminum baking
  powder
1/2 teaspoon each cinnamon and
  ground coriander

3 tablespoons sugar
2 tablespoons unhulled sesame seeds
  (see Notes)
1 large egg
1/4 cup peanut oil
2 tablespoons frozen pineapple or
  apple juice concentrate
1/2 cup evaporated skim milk
3/4 cup water
1/2 cup raisins

1. Preheat oven to 400 degrees. Sift first 6 listed ingredients into a large bowl. Stir in sugar and sesame seeds.
2. In another bowl, combine egg, oil, and concentrate. Blend with fork. Pour milk and water into a 2-cup measure.
3. Make a well in center of dry ingredients. Add egg mixture and stir only until dry mixture is moistened. While stirring, add milk, a little at a time. Fold in raisins.
4. Grease 12 3-inch muffin cups lightly with sweet butter/margarine blend. Fill each cup three-quarters full. Bake for 20 minutes, or until muffins are lightly brown and dough pulls away from sides of cups. Place pan on rack and let stand for 3 minutes. Loosen around sides with blunt knife. Remove muffins and let cool on rack for 2 minutes before serving.

Yield: **12 muffins**

Variation: For blueberry-buckwheat muffins, rinse and pick over 1 cup fresh blueberries. Drain well. To above recipe, add 1/2 teaspoon grated lemon zest and 1 tablespoon honey in Step 2. Fold berries into batter at end of Step 3 in place of raisins. If desired, dust with confectioner's sugar while warm.

Notes:

1. Buckwheat flour and unhulled sesame seeds are available in health-food stores.
2. Freeze muffins wrapped in foil, and reheat in foil in a preheated 400-degree oven for about 15 minutes.

BANANA-OAT MUFFINS

1 1/2 cups unbleached flour
2 1/2 teaspoons non-aluminum
　baking powder
1/2 cup rolled oats
1/4 cup unprocessed bran
1/2 teaspoon ground ginger
2 tablespoons tightly packed brown
　sugar or date powder (see
　Notes)
2 1/2 tablespoons pure unsalted

peanut butter
2 tablespoons flavorful honey
1/2 cup unsweetened pineapple juice
2 tablespoons each peanut oil and
　melted sweet butter/margarine
　blend
3/4 cup evaporated skim milk
1 large egg
1 ripe banana, cut into 1/4-inch
　pieces

1. Preheat oven to 375 degrees. Sift flour and baking powder into a large bowl. Stir in oats, bran, ginger, and sugar or date powder.
2. Place peanut butter in small cereal bowl. Spoon with honey and mash. Stir in juice. Add oil and shortening and blend.
3. Pour milk into a measuring cup. Add egg and beat lightly with fork. Make a well in the center of the dry ingredients. Stir in peanut butter mixture and stir only until dry ingredients are moistened. While stirring, add milk mix gradually.
4. Grease 12 3-inch muffin cups lightly with sweet butter/margarine blend. Fill each cup with equal amounts of batter. Push proportional amount of banana pieces into each batter-filled cup. Bake for 23 to 25 minutes, or until lightly brown. Place pan on rack for 5 minutes. With blunt knife, loosen each muffin around sides. Gently lift out of cups and place on rack. Serve warm.

Yield: 12 muffins

Notes:

1. Date powder (also called date sugar) is a good sugar substitute. It's simply dried dates that have been finely chopped; no sugar is added. Use it also to sprinkle over dry and cooked cereals, fruit, and puddings. It's generally available in health-food stores.
2. Freeze muffins wrapped in foil, and reheat in foil in a preheated 400-degree oven for about 15 minutes.

POP-MUFFINS

3/4 cup plus 2 tablespoons
  unbleached flour
1/4 teaspoon salt
1/2 teaspoon cinnamon
1/4 teaspoon ground coriander
1/2 teaspoon sugar
2 tablespoons oat bran; pulverized
1 tablespoon regular wheat germ
2 large eggs

3/4 cup milk (preferably 1% milk
  fat)
1/4 cup low-fat buttermilk,
  preferably unsalted
1 tablespoon sweet
  butter/margarine blend,
  melted
2 tablespoons unhulled sesame seeds

1. Preheat oven to 425 degrees. Put all the flour, salt, and spices into a large bowl. Stir in sugar, oat bran, and wheat germ.
2. Drop eggs into food blender. Add milks and whir on high speed for 1 minute. Whisk into dry ingredients until well blended. Stir in melted shortening. Let stand for 1 minute.
3. Grease seven 5-ounce pottery crocks or glass custard cups with sweet butter/margarine blend. Sprinkle the bottom of each cup with a thin layer of sesame seeds. Place cups in large shallow baking pan. Fill each cup two-thirds full with batter. Bake for 20 minutes. Reduce heat to 375 degrees (do not open oven door). Bake for 18 minutes longer. Cut small slits into sides of each muffin. Continue baking for 2 minutes.
4. Remove from oven. Circle each cup carefully with a blunt knife to loosen. Gently lift out muffins. Serve hot.

Yield: **7 large pop-muffins**

Variation: To make cheese pop-muffins, sprinkle each cupful of batter with 1 teaspoon freshly grated Parmesan cheese before baking.

Serving suggestions: For breakfast: Split and fill muffin with Curried Scrambled Eggs (see Menu Plan, page 217) or low-fat cottage cheese and fruit juice–sweetened jelly. For lunch: Split and fill with Lump Crabmeat Sauce (page 150).

Note: Muffins taste best fresh from the oven.

11

SALADS AND SALAD DRESSINGS

MIXED SALAD WITH CARROT JUICE VINAIGRETTE

Sweet crisp carrots in the salad and sweet smooth carrot juice in the dressing are paired in a refreshing mixed salad. A lovely low-calorie way to start a meal or accompany such main courses as Oven-"Fried" Chicken, Pork Chops with Fennel, or Skewered Monkfish (pages 74, 143, 122).

1/4 cup unseasoned fresh or canned carrot juice
3 tablespoons balsamic vinegar
1/2 teaspoon dry mustard
3 tablespoons Italian olive oil
1 tablespoon fresh lemon juice
1/2 teaspoon dried tarragon leaves, crumbled
1 small crisp green head romaine lettuce, tough center section

removed, torn into bite-size pieces
1 small carrot, peeled and grated or shredded
1/3 cup coarsely chopped red onion
2 tablespoons coarsely chopped fresh coriander
2 tablespoons raisins (optional)
1/4 teaspoons salt
Freshly ground black pepper

1. In a small bowl, whisk together carrot juice, vinegar, mustard, oil, and lemon juice. Whisk in tarragon. Let stand while salad is prepared.

2. Rinse and dry romaine well before tearing into pieces. Then place it in a salad bowl with carrot, onion, and coriander. Pour dressing over mixture, tossing to coat. Stir in raisins if desired. Sprinkle with salt and toss gently again. Serve freshly ground pepper on the side.

Yield: **Serves 4 to 5; 1/2 cup dressing**

SAFFRON RICE SALAD WITH RED PEPPER SAUCE

When pasta salad palls, cook rice in my enriched stock, and enrobe it with a saffron-scented purée of red peppers. Serve it as a side dish, or top with morsels of cooked-and-chilled fish, meat, or poultry for a luncheon main course.

3 large sweet red peppers
About 1 cup each Chicken Stock (page 19) or Vegetable Stock (page 20), and water
2 teaspoons Savory Seasoning (page 15)
¾ cup rice
3 tablespoons Italian olive oil
1 tablespoon cider vinegar
1½ teaspoons prepared Dijon mustard, preferably unsalted
¼ teaspoon salt
⅛ teaspoon freshly ground black pepper
½ teaspoon whole saffron threads, soaked in 2 teaspoons boiling water
1 large Kirby cucumber, peeled, cut into ¼-inch pieces
1 small red onion, coarsely chopped (about ½ cup)
2 tablespoons minced Italian flat parsley
Crisp lettuce leaves
Radish rosettes

1. Char peppers first. Preheat broiler. Place peppers on rack in broiling pan 3 inches from heat and blacken all over. Transfer to plastic bag and seal. Let stand 15 minutes to steam. Peel off skins (they'll slip right off), catching juices in bowl underneath. Cut each pepper in half and seed. Slice one pepper into ¼-inch strips and set aside. Cut remaining peppers into chunks.

2. In 1¾-quart heavy-bottomed saucepan bring stock and water to a boil. Add Savory Seasoning and rice. Bring to a boil again. Stir, then cover tightly. Reduce heat and simmer until cooked but still firm. If liquid evaporates before done, add a bit more stock, re-cover, and continue cooking a few minutes longer (all liquid should be absorbed). Turn into a bowl and let cool for 15 minutes, separating rice with fork.

3. Place pepper chunks in bowl of a food processor that has been fitted with a steel knife. Add oil, vinegar, mustard, salt, and pepper. Purée until very smooth. Add saffron and liquid and purée for 3 seconds.

4. Pour purée over rice, stirring to combine. Then add cucumber,

onion, and parsley. Gently fold in reserved pepper strips. Cover and let stand at room temperature for 30 minutes. Stir just before serving.

5. Arrange lettuce in one layer on decorative platter. Serve salad over lettuce. Garnish with radish rosettes.

Yield: **Serves 6**

Note: Sauce (recipe through Step 3) doubles as a dip for boiled or sautéed shrimp. Try it, too, with skewered barbecued chicken or meat.

WATERCRESS AND MUSHROOM SALAD

Tender mushrooms and peppery watercress combine with crisp sprouts for an enticingly textured salad. The dressing is good with any combination of vegetable salad ingredients.

3 tablespoons each Chicken Stock (page 19) or Vegetable Stock (page 20), Italian olive oil, and red wine vinegar
1/2 teaspoon prepared dried Dijon mustard, preferably without salt
1 teaspoon Savory Seasoning (page 15)
1 bunch crisp watercress, tough stems removed, rinsed and dried
1/4 pound snow-white fresh mushrooms, ends trimmed, damp-wiped and thin-sliced
1 teaspoon minced garlic
1/2 cup alfalfa sprouts
1/4 teaspoon salt
Freshly ground black pepper

1. In a small bowl, whisk together stock, oil, vinegar, mustard, and Savory Seasoning. Let mixture stand while salad is prepared.

2. Put watercress, mushrooms, and garlic in a salad bowl. Toss with half the dressing. Then add sprouts, pulling them apart to distribute evenly. Sprinkle with salt and remaining dressing. Toss briefly.

3. Serve on individual plates, sprinkled with pepper to taste.

Yield: **Serves 4; about 1/2 cup dressing**

SAVOY SALAD

Pungent Savoy cabbage is mingled with sweet green pepper, onion, and pimentos for a cole slaw that's gone to gourmet cooking school.

1 medium Savoy cabbage
1 medium sweet green pepper
1 medium onion
2 teaspoons superfine sugar
1/4 teaspoon each salt and freshly
    ground black pepper
1 cup loosely packed fresh dill,
    coarsely chopped
2 unsalted pimentos, drained,
    coarsely chopped

2 tablespoons fresh lemon juice
About 2 teaspoons prepared Dijon
    mustard, preferably without
    salt
1 tablespoon rice wine vinegar
1 tablespoon frozen pineapple juice
    concentrate
2/3 cup low-fat unsalted buttermilk
1/2 cup Light Choice sour cream
Dill sprigs

1. Cut cabbage into wedges to fit food processor feed tube. Set shredding attachment in place in workbowl. Fine-shred cabbage, using light pressure. Measure out 4 cups. Scrape into large bowl.
2. Fit food processor with steel blade. Cut pepper and onion into 2-inch pieces; add to workbowl. Fine-chop in on/off turns. Add to bowl. Sprinkle with sugar, salt, and pepper, stirring to blend. Fold in dill and pimentos.
3. In a small bowl, whisk lemon juice, mustard, vinegar, and concentrate. Pour over salad and combine. Shake container of buttermilk (it tends to be thick), measure out, and combine with salad. Fold in sour cream. Mixture will be very moist.
4. Pile equal amounts of solids and liquid into 2 quart-size jars, turning jars upside down from time to time to distribute juices. Chill for 2 hours. To serve, drain off most of liquid with slotted spoon and transfer salad to decorative bowl, reserving juices to store leftovers. Garnish with dill sprigs.

Yield: **1 quart**

Serving suggestion: Drain and serve this salad on meat or poultry sandwiches in place of lettuce or tomato.

WARM RADICCHIO SALAD

Radicchio (pronounced ra-DEEK-kyoh) is the generic name for a group of red chicory. Here, radicchio leaves are given a quick under-the-broiler cooking (to blunt their bitterness), then filled with well-seasoned vegetables and cheese.

3 tablespoons Italian olive oil
1 bunch scallions (8 medium),
  using white section and some
  of tender green stems, coarsely
  chopped
1 small sweet red pepper, seeded,
  coarsely chopped
1 tablespoon Savory Seasoning
  (page 15)
1 medium Golden Delicious apple,
  peeled, cut into ½-inch cubes
½ cup coarsely chopped seeded ripe
  tomato
2 tablespoons plus 1½ teaspoons
  raspberry or red wine vinegar
1 teaspoon prepared Dijon
  mustard, preferably without
  salt
⅛ to ¼ teaspoon salt
2 light dashes cayenne pepper
1 teaspoon Worcestershire sauce
¼ cup grated part-skim mozzarella
2 tablespoons mashed ripe avocado
  pear (optional)

1. Heat 2 tablespoons oil in nonstick skillet. Sauté scallions and pepper for 2 minutes over moderate heat. Sprinkle with seasoning. Combine apple and tomato with mixture. Sauté over medium-high heat for 1 minute.
2. Push ingredients to center of skillet. Pour 2 tablespoons vinegar around sides of skillet. Cook, without stirring, for 30 seconds; combine ingredients.
3. Stir in mustard, salt, cayenne pepper, and Worcestershire sauce. Cook for 30 seconds. Remove from heat. Blend in mozzarella and avocado, if desired. Set aside. Preheat broiler.
4. Separate radicchio leaves. Set out 4 individual gratinée dishes. Overlap edges of 3 leaves in each dish. Combine remaining 1 tablespoon oil with 1½ teaspoons vinegar. Brush over leaves. Place under broiler for 1 minute. Spread immediately with equal portions of filling. Serve warm.

Yield: **Serves 4**

LENTIL/BULGUR SALAD WITH FRUIT AND VEGETABLES

This is a colorful, substantial entree like no other salad you've ever tasted.

½ cup brown lentils
½ cup bulgur
1 tablespoon frozen apple juice
  concentrate
2 cups water
1 tablespoon Savory Seasoning
  (page 15)
½ teaspoon mild curry powder
small Bouquet Garni (page 16)
2 tablespoons fresh lime juice
1 tablespoon cider vinegar
2 teaspoons prepared Dijon
  mustard, preferably without
  salt

¼ teaspoon salt
3 tablespoons Italian olive oil
6 large scallions, including tender
  green section
1 small sweet red pepper, seeded,
  cut into ¼-inch strips
¼ cup coarsely chopped parsley or
  fresh coriander
1 large navel orange, cut into
  1-inch chunks (see Notes)
Crisp greens (e.g. arugula,
  romaine, watercress)
Freshly ground black pepper

1. Put lentils in strainer. Pick over, then rinse under cold running water for 1 minute. Drain. Place in bowl. Cover with cold water and let soak for 1 hour. Drain. Add fresh water. Repeat procedure once more. Soak for 2 hours (see Notes). Drain.
2. Put bulgur in 1-cup measure. Fill with water. Let stand for 5 minutes. Drain off small amount of water. Set aside.
3. In 1½-quart heavy-bottomed saucepan, combine lentils, concentrate, water, seasonings, and bouquet garni. Bring to a boil. Reduce heat. Cover and simmer for 20 minutes. Add bulgur. Raise heat and slow-boil, uncovered, for 5 minutes. Pour into strainer. Discard bouquet garni. Let drain until cool. Transfer to salad bowl.
4. In a small bowl, whisk lime juice with vinegar, mustard, salt, and oil, blending well. Let stand for 5 minutes. Whisk again. Pour over salad and stir gently. Using 2 large spoons, carefully fold in scallions, red pepper, and coriander; then fold in orange. Let stand at room temperature for 30 minutes before serving, stirring once midway. Or refrigerate, bringing to room temperature before serving.

5. Mound on crisp greens and sprinkle with pepper to taste.

Yield: **About 4½ cups; serves 6 to 7**

Notes:

1. If recipe is prepared early in the day, carefully fold in orange 30 minutes before serving.
2. I've recently observed that the tenderness of lentils varies with each bag. If you notice that they begin to fall apart during the second soaking, drain, rinse under cold running water, and use promptly.

BOK CHOY SALAD

Crisp, bittersweet bok choy is combined here with sweet carrot, zesty red onion, and leaf lettuce and dressed with a walnut oil dressing.

Small head green leaf lettuce (tough center sections removed), rinsed and well-dried
1 cup ½-inch strips fresh bok choy
⅓ cup shredded carrot
1 medium red onion, thinly sliced, separated into rings

2 tablespoons coarsely chopped fresh parsley or fresh mint leaves
1 recipe Buttermilk Salad Dressing (page 180)
4 to 6 large radishes, cut into rosettes

1. Break lettuce into bite-size pieces and place in large bowl. Add next 4 ingredients and toss gently.
2. Pour dressing over salad just before serving, tossing to coat. Arrange on individual salad plates, each serving topped with a radish.

Yield: **Serves 4 to 6**

FRESH BEET AND POTATO SALAD

I use the delicious stems and leaves of the beet to enhance flavor and fiber in beet dishes. So shop for crisp stems, small tender leaves, and firm beets. I bake the beets in their jackets to seal in flavor and nutrients, and quickly boil the stems and leaves, which I combine with the salad.

1 bunch fresh beets with leaves (3 to 4 medium beets)
1 pound Idaho potatoes, cut into ½-inch cubes

1 medium red onion, halved and thinly sliced
6 tablespoons Garlic Dressing (page 181)

1. Cut stems from beets. Rinse well. Pull leaves off stems. Break stems every 2 inches, peeling back strings. Drop leaves and stems into a potful of boiling water. Boil for 5 minutes. Drain in colander, then on sheet of paper toweling. Slice into 1-inch pieces. Place in a large bowl. Preheat oven to 400 degrees.
2. Wash beets. Dry off and wrap tightly in aluminum foil. Bake for 1 to 1½ hours, testing with point of knife after 1 hour. Remove from foil and let cool until easy to handle. Peel off skins; cut into ⅜-inch slices. Place in a large bowl.
3. Cook potatoes in medium heavy-bottomed saucepan in water to cover until firm-tender (about 12 minutes). Drain in colander and let cool. Add to beets. Break up onion into rings and add to bowl.
4. Pour just-whisked dressing over salad, and combine carefully with 2 large spoons.

Yield: **About 4½ cups; serves 6**

Variations: Sprinkle in 2 tablespoons freshly grated Parmesan cheese or stir in 1 tablespoon prepared beet horseradish just before serving.

BUTTERMILK DRESSING

Sharp horseradish and Dijon mustard are tempered with buttermilk in this smooth salad dressing.

¼ cup walnut oil
2 tablespoons wine vinegar
2 teaspoons white wine
    Worcestershire sauce
1 tablespoon Savory Seasoning
    (page 15)

Pinch salt
1 teaspoon each prepared white
    horseradish and Dijon
    mustard
3 tablespoons low-fat buttermilk,
    preferably without salt

1. Pour oil into small bowl. Whisk in vinegar, Worcestershire sauce, and seasonings. Let stand for 5 minutes.
2. Combine horseradish with mustard. Whisk into dressing; stir in buttermilk. Use immediately.

Yield: **About ½ cup**

GARLIC DRESSING

For more than three thousand years, folklore has extolled the medicinal virtues of garlic. I've been extolling the health-promoting features of this tasty herb since I published *The Dieter's Gourmet Cookbook* in 1979. Chinese scientists now identify garlic (as well as its related alliums such as onions, scallions, and Chinese chives) as a weapon in the war against bacterial infections and cancer (*The New York Times,* January 1, 1989). I've developed a new way to cook garlic so it can be used in a salad dressing as a mild flavor-enhancer. Now you can take your medicine and like it!

6 large cloves garlic, peeled and
    halved
½ cup Vegetable Stock (page 20)
    or Chicken Stock (page 19)
½ teaspoon finely minced lemon
    zest
2 tablespoons rice wine vinegar
1 tablespoon red wine vinegar

¼ cup fresh orange juice
1½ tablespoons fresh lemon juice
¼ teaspoon each salt, dry
    mustard, and mild curry
    powder
1½ tablespoons Italian olive oil
1 tablespoon finely minced parsley
Black pepper to taste

1. Place garlic in small enameled saucepan with stock. Bring to a boil. Reduce heat, cover partially, and simmer until all liquid evaporates (8 to 10 minutes); avoid scorching. Transfer garlic to small bowl and mash.
2. Whisk in remaining ingredients. Let stand for 5 minutes. Whisk again just before pouring over salad.

Yield: **About ⅔ cup**

SPICY LOW-CHOLESTEROL MAYONNAISE

My mayonnaise uses fifty percent less fat than commercial or home-made mayonnaise. I've blended a mere ½ egg yolk into a mixture of oil and high-protein tofu. Spiked with sharp horseradish, curry, and mustard, it makes a wonderful mayonnaise for every health-minded person.

¾ cup mashed tofu, drained and
  dried
Pinch cayenne pepper
2 tablespoons wine vinegar
1½ teaspoons prepared unsalted
  Dijon mustard
½ teaspoon superfine sugar
½ teaspoon dried tarragon leaves,
  crumbled
½ egg yolk

¼ teaspoon salt
½ teaspoon mild curry powder
½ cup Italian olive oil or peanut
  oil
2 tablespoons minced parsley
1½ tablespoons Light Choice sour
  cream
1 teaspoon prepared white
  horseradish

1. Fit food processor with steel blade. Put tofu in workbowl. Add cayenne pepper, 1 tablespoon vinegar, and ½ teaspoon mustard, sugar, and tarragon. Process until smooth and well blended. Set aside.
2. In a small bowl, place egg yolk, salt, remaining 1 teaspoon mustard, curry powder, remaining 1 tablespoon vinegar, and 1 tablespoon oil. Using wire whisk, beat until well blended. While whisking, slowly drizzle in ¼ cup oil in a steady *thin* stream until mixture thickens. Whisk for 30 seconds without adding more oil. Then add remaining oil, a tablespoon at a time, whisking after each addition. Mayonnaise will become very thick.
3. Scrape into workbowl with tofu. Add parsley. Process for 20 seconds until smooth and well blended. Remove steel blade, scraping off any clinging mayonnaise into workbowl. Stir in sour cream and horseradish.
4. Spoon into glass jar and refrigerate. Mixture thickens to a firmer texture when chilled.

Yield: **1 cup**

Variations:

1. Substitute minced chives for parsley, and use 1 tablespoon each lemon juice and tarragon vinegar in place of wine vinegar.
2. Substitute ¼ teaspoon freshly ground white or black pepper for cayenne pepper.

Note: I find that by hand-whisking the egg and oil first and then combining them with puréed tofu in the food processor, I get a better cohesion of ingredients.

RUSSIAN TARTAR SAUCE

Inspired by Russian dressing and Tartar sauce, this is a condiment for mayonnaise lovers who could do with less fat and cholesterol. There's only ¼ teaspoon of mayonnaise in each teaspoon of this sauce.

¼ cup good-quality commercial mayonnaise
1 teaspoon Italian olive oil
½ teaspoon mild curry powder
3 tablespoons fresh lemon juice
4 teaspoons each unsalted tomato paste and prepared Dijon mustard, preferably without

salt
2 teaspoons wine vinegar
½ cup Light Choice sour cream
2 tablespoons minced flat Italian parsley, or 1 tablespoon each parsley and minced chives
2 tablespoons minced shallot

1. Place mayonnaise and oil in a small bowl. Blend with wire whisk.
2. In a cup, combine curry powder, lemon juice, tomato paste, mustard, and vinegar, whisking to blend. Whisk into mayonnaise mixture. Stir in remaining ingredients.
3. Spoon into glass jar. Cover tightly and refrigerate for at least 2 hours before using.

Yield: **About 1 cup**

12

SWEETS

SAUTÉED FRUIT WITH TOASTED ALMONDS

Two fruit staples, apples and bananas, are no longer as naturally sweet as they used to be. But they are now—quick-sautéed with spices and just a soupçon of sweetener. A breeze to make and a delight to eat.

3 tablespoons sliced almonds, blanched
1 tablespoon sweet butter/margarine blend
¼ teaspoon each ground ginger, ground coriander, and cinnamon
1 teaspoon superfine sugar

2 Golden Delicious apples, peeled, cored, and thin-sliced
2 almost-ripe large bananas, cut into ¼-inch slices
1 tablespoon flavorful honey, such as thyme
2 tablespoons dry sherry
½ lemon

1. Spread almonds across a large nonstick skillet. Over low heat, toast to golden brown, shaking skillet often and adjusting heat when necessary to prevent scorching. Transfer to dish.
2. Add shortening to skillet. Over medium-high heat, cook until bubbly. Sprinkle in spices and sugar. Cook for 15 seconds.
3. Arrange apples in one layer across skillet. Sauté for 1 minute without stirring. Stir and cook for 1 minute longer. Add bananas and combine. Sauté, stirring gently from time to time, until fruit begins to soften (about 4 minutes). Dribble honey over mixture; squeeze juice from ½ lemon over all.
4. Spoon onto warm individual serving dishes, sprinkled with toasted almonds.

Yield: **Serves 4**

Serving suggestion: Top with Light Raspberry/Banana Ice Cream or Raspberry/Chocolate Sauce (pages 206 or 208).

DELICATE APPLE/CRANBERRY PIE

A crunchy yet paper-thin crust envelopes a mélange of juicy Golden Delicious apples, tart fresh cranberries, spices, and just enough sugar. I've used fifty percent less flour, sugar, and saturated fat than that used in traditional fruit pies without sacrificing flavor or texture. The crust freezes successfully; and, defrosted within one hour, it rolls out with little effort to smooth perfection.

For the pastry:

1/4 cup rolled oats
1 cup unbleached flour, spooned into measuring cup and leveled off with knife
1/4 teaspoon salt
1/2 teaspoon non-aluminum baking powder

1/4 teaspoon each ground coriander and cinnamon
1 teaspoon sugar
2 tablespoons each peanut oil and melted sweet butter/margarine blend, combined
4 to 5 tablespoons hot tap water

For the filling:

1 tablespoon frozen orange juice concentrate
2 teaspoons fresh lemon juice
1/2 teaspoon finely minced lemon zest
5 large Golden Delicious apples, quartered, cored, peeled, and thinly sliced
1/2 cup fresh cranberries, rinsed and drained
6 tablespoons sugar

1/2 teaspoon each cinnamon and freshly grated nutmeg
2 cloves, crushed, or 1/4 teaspoon ground cardamom
4 to 5 teaspoons quick-cooking tapioca (see Notes)
1 tablespoon sweet butter/margarine blend, cut into small pieces
1 tablespoon milk
1 teaspoon superfine sugar

1. Preheat oven to 425 degrees. To prepare pastry, fit food processor with steel blade. Place oats in workbowl and pulverize. Add flour, salt, baking powder, spices, and sugar. Process for 10 seconds. With machine running, pour oil mixture slowly through feed tube. Process for 6 seconds. Then spoon hot water through feed tube. Process until dough forms soft balls that rotate in workbowl 4 or 5 times. Dough

should be pliable but not sticky. If sticky, sprinkle with a teaspoon additional flour and process for 3 seconds.

2. Scoop up dough and shape into 2 balls. Lay each ball on a sheet of wax paper. Press each piece gently into a flat 8-inch circle; wrap each circle separately in plastic film and chill for 30 minutes. (May be made a day ahead, refrigerated, and rolled out after returning to room temperature.)

3. To roll out pastry, moisten rolling surface. Place a large sheet of wax paper on surface. Place 1 circle of dough on paper and cover with another sheet of wax paper. Roll dough gently between both sheets of paper to a 12-inch circle. (Dough will be very thin.) Remove top sheet of paper gingerly; lift up bottom sheet with dough and invert onto an 8-inch pie pan, pressing around sides. Peel paper by tearing down center first and then peeling each half toward sides of pan.

4. To prepare filling, combine concentrate, lemon juice, and lemon zest in a large bowl. Add apples, turning to coat. Stir in cranberries.

5. In a small bowl, combine sugar, spices, and tapioca. Sprinkle over fruit, stirring to coat evenly. Fill crust with mixture, mounding in center, making certain that apples are spread to sides. Strew with shortening.

6. Roll out the top crust following directions in Step 2. Lay loosely over pie, then peel off paper carefully, moving from center outward. Trim pastry ½ inch beyond edge of pan. Press both crusts together and turn under, pushing against pan. Crimp edges with fork. Again with fork, poke several holes in top crust.

7. Position rack in lower section of oven. Bake pie for 15 minutes. Reduce heat to 375 degrees and bake for 25 minutes longer. (If crust browns too rapidly, cover loosely with sheet of aluminum foil.) Brush with milk and sprinkle with sugar. Return to oven for 5 to 8 minutes, until crust is delicately browned. Remove from oven, place on rack, and let cool for 45 minutes. Serve warm.

Yield: **One 8-inch pie; serves 8**

Notes:

1. If apples are particularly juicy, use 5 teaspoons of tapioca.
2. Fully baked crust will be delicately browned and crispy. For a paler crust, reduce baking time by 5 minutes.

OATMEAL CHIP COOKIES WITH APRICOTS

Apricot puree tops these chewy-centered, crisp-edged cookies. They use less sugars and fats than traditional oatmeal cookies, deriving their delightful texture and special sweetness from fruit juice concentrate and sweet spices instead.

4 ounces dried unsulphured apricots
2 tablespoons flavorful honey, such as thyme
1½ cups unbleached flour
½ teaspoon each non-aluminum baking powder, baking soda, and salt
1 teaspoon each ground cardamom and cinnamon
5 tablespoons sweet butter/margarine blend, plus up to 1 teaspoon for cookie

sheets
3 tablespoons peanut oil
½ cup firmly packed light brown sugar (not granulated)
2 tablespoons granulated sugar
3 tablespoons frozen apple juice concentrate
1 large egg
1½ cups 1-minute quick oats
1½ teaspoons pure vanilla extract
2 tablespoons unsalted buttermilk
½ cup coarsely chopped walnuts
½ cup unsweetened carob chips

1. Put apricots in colander. Rinse under cold running water. Transfer to a small enameled saucepan. Add just enough water to cover. Let soak for 10 minutes. Place over high heat. Bring to a boil. Reduce heat to a slow boil and cook, uncovered, stirring from time to time until most of liquid is evaporated and fruit is soft. (One cup of mixture should remain in saucepan.) Stir in honey; let cool for 5 minutes. Purée in food processor or blender. Transfer to cup and set aside. (May be made a day ahead and refrigerated in a tightly closed jar.)

2. Preheat oven to 375 degrees. Sift flour, baking powder, baking soda, salt, and spices into bowl.

3. Place 5 tablespoons shortening, oil, and sugars in a large mixing machine bowl. Beat on medium speed until well blended. Scrape down sides of bowl. Add concentrate and beat for 30 seconds. Drop egg into mixture, beating until light and fluffy. Scrape down sides of bowl.

4. Add oats and vanilla extract. Beat on medium speed for 30 seconds. With machine running, gradually add flour mix. Then combine buttermilk and walnuts with mixture and beat for 30 seconds. Stir or beat in carob chips.

5. Drop dough by teaspoonsful onto cookie sheets that have been lightly greased with remaining shortening, arranging about 16 cookies on each sheet in rows of 4. With moistened fork, flatten dough to ¼-inch thickness. Shape into 2-inch circles. Bake in center section of oven for exactly 8 minutes.

6. With a small spoon, make a depression in the center of each cookie. Fill each with ¾ teaspoon apricot puree. Return to oven until lightly browned (5 to 5½ minutes; do not overbake). Using a spatula, transfer to wire rack. (Cookies are slightly soft when warm, but they crisp up when cooled.) After baking day, pack cookies loosely in sturdy plastic containers and store in freezer.

Yield: **About 45 cookies**

Variation: One-third cup chocolate chips can be substituted for carob chips.

Note: Unsulphured apricots and unsweetened carob chips are generally available in health-food stores.

ANGELIC SPONGE CAKE

Angel food cake is the prescribed baked dessert for cholesterol/fat watchers because it rates zero in both those ingredients. But it's pretty bland in texture and taste (unless you're thrilled by massive overdoses of sugar).

Sponge cake, on the other hand, is traditionally made with 6 to 9 egg yolks—a heavy cargo of cholesterol/fat—but is as richly flavored as it is textured. So I've incorporated angel food cake techniques into a sponge cake that tastes traditional but has only three 3 yolks. The cholesterol/fat content per serving is quite low, and so is the sugar. My Angelic Sponge Cake is a heavenly alternative to angel food cake.

1 cup cake flour (not self-rising), sifted before measuring
1/4 teaspoon each salt and freshly grated nutmeg
1/2 teaspoon ground ginger
1 1/2 teaspoons non-aluminum baking powder
1/2 cup superfine sugar

9 large eggs at room temperature (use 3 yolks and 9 whites)
1 large lemon
1 tablespoon frozen orange juice concentrate
1/4 teaspoon almond extract
1/2 teaspoon pure vanilla extract
1/4 teaspoon cream of tartar

1. Preheat oven to 350 degrees. Sift flour, salt, spices, and baking powder 3 times (2 sheets of wax paper work well). Transfer gently to a bowl. Sift sugar 3 times onto separate sheets of wax paper and finally into a cup. Set aside.
2. Separate eggs, dropping 3 yolks into a medium bowl and 9 whites into the large bowl of mixing machine.
3. Using swivel-bladed vegetable peeler, peel zest from lemon, taking care not to include any of the bitter white pith. Fine-chop zest by hand, or mince in an electric herb chopper. Measure out 2 teaspoons and add to egg yolks. Cut lemon in half and squeeze 1 teaspoon juice into yolks. By hand, whisk in concentrate, 1/4 cup sugar, and extracts. Gently stir in 1/4 cup flour mixture.
4. Using whisk attachment of mixing machine, beat egg whites on medium speed until foamy. Increase speed and slowly add remaining 1/4 cup sugar and cream of tartar. Beat on highest speed until glossy and stiff.
5. Using wooden spoon, stir about 1/3 cup beaten egg whites into yolk mixture. Then scrape all of yolk mixture back into remaining beaten egg whites, combining both using a folding motion 4 times. Carefully fold in remaining flour mix.

6. Spoon into an ungreased 9-inch tube pan, smoothing out top. Run spatula around sides of batter and tube to release air bubbles. Place in center section of oven and bake for 10 minutes. Reduce heat to 325 degrees and bake for 30 to 35 minutes longer. Check after 30 minutes. Finished cake should be lightly browned and spring back when top is pressed lightly.

7. Remove pan from oven and invert. (A 3-cup mason jar with a 2½-inch neck will hold the tube.) Let cake cool completely (about 1½ hours). Run sharp knife around sides of pan and tube to unmold. To serve, cut cake with sharp serrated knife.

Yield: **12 servings**

Note: Cake freezes well if stored in plastic wrap that is then covered with aluminum foil. Take care that there is no pressure put against it while freezing. Pieces can be cut off while still frozen; they'll defrost rapidly at room temperature.

APPLE-FILLED COFFEE CAKE

Thin-sliced Golden Delicious apples, dipped in lemon juice and honey, are interspersed between layers of light-textured batter and baked to a crusty brown.

1 tablespoon flavorful honey
2 tablespoons fresh lemon juice
2 large Golden Delicious apples, peeled, cored, quartered, thinly sliced lengthwise
1 1/2 cups unbleached flour
1/2 teaspoon baking soda
2 teaspoons non-aluminum baking powder
1/4 cup oat bran
5 tablespoons sweet butter/margarine blend

1/4 cup tightly packed dark brown sugar
1 1/2 teaspoons pure vanilla extract
2 eggs, separated
1/2 cup each low-fat plain yogurt and Light Choice sour cream
6 teaspoons granulated sugar
1/4 teaspoon each ground cardamom and freshly grated nutmeg
1 teaspoon cinnamon
1 teaspoon confectioner's sugar

1. Preheat oven to 350 degrees. Spoon honey into medium bowl. While stirring, add lemon juice until blended. Drop apples into bowl as they're cut, turning often to coat. Set aside.
2. Sift flour, baking soda, and baking powder onto a sheet of wax paper. Sprinkle with bran and combine.
3. In large bowl of mixing machine, beat shortening with brown sugar and vanilla extract at high speed until well blended. Scrape down sides of bowl. Add egg yolks. Beat on medium speed for 1 minute. Scrape down sides of bowl. Combine yogurt and sour cream. Form flour-covered wax paper into a funnel and, on medium speed, beat in dry ingredients alternately with yogurt mix. Then beat on medium-high speed until light and fluffy.
4. In mixing machine bowl, beat egg whites at moderate speed until foamy. While beating at high speed, sprinkle in 4 teaspoons granulated sugar. Beat on high speed until glossy and firm. Stir 1/4 beaten mix into batter; fold in remainder.
5. In a cup, combine remaining 2 teaspoons granulated sugar with spices. Grease a 9-inch loose-bottomed tube pan with sweet butter-margarine blend. Spoon half the batter into pan, spreading out evenly. Arrange half the apple slices on batter in one layer. Sprinkle

with half the spice mix. Cover apples evenly with remaining batter. Arrange residual apples in a neat pattern on batter, pressing gently into cake. Sprinkle apples with leftover spice mix. Pour half the juices from apples over all.

6. Bake in center section of oven for 50 minutes. Place pan on rack. Sprinkle cake with confectioner's sugar. Let cool in pan for 10 minutes. With blunt knife, loosen around sides of pan and lift out tube. Place on rack for 15 minutes. Then gently loosen around tube and bottom of pan, and carefully transfer to rack. Cool to room temperature before placing on serving dish. Cut wedges with sharp serrated knife.

Yield: **Serves 8 to 10**

Note: To maintain taste and texture, foil-wrap leftovers and freeze. Reheat in preheated 400-degree oven for 15 to 20 minutes.

TUTTI-FRUTTI CHIFFON PIE

Crunchy-crusted, with a filling that's feather-light, this is a delicious finale to any meal. Actually, you can have two finales, because it's so light your scale won't notice the second portion! And it will keep nicely in your fridge for two days.

For the crust:

1 cup Nutri-Grain biscuits or spoon-size shredded wheat
1/4 cup regular wheat germ
1/2 teaspoon each ground coriander and cinnamon
2/3 cup plus 1 tablespoon fine graham cracker crumbs (see Note)
2 tablespoons each melted sweet butter/margarine blend and peanut oil, combined
3 tablespoons ice water

For the filling:

1 8-ounce can unsweetened pineapple tidbits, or chunks cut into small pieces
2 tablespoons frozen orange juice concentrate
1 tablespoon fresh lemon juice
1/2 teaspoon freshly grated nutmeg
2 packages plain gelatin
2 large eggs, separated (use 1 yolk and 2 whites)
2 tablespoons each sugar and flavorful honey
1 10-ounce box frozen sliced strawberries in syrup, partially defrosted
3/4 cup unsalted dry-curd cottage cheese (1/2% milk fat)
1/3 cup evaporated skim milk

1. To prepare crust, place first 3 listed ingredients in workbowl of food processor that has been fitted with a steel blade. Process to a fine-crumb consistency. Add graham cracker crumbs to mix.
2. With machine running, pour shortening mix through feed tube. Process for 8 seconds. Then, with machine still running, pour in water, 1 tablespoon at a time, and process until mixture congeals and forms large chunks. Scrape into an 8-inch pie pan. With fingers, press evenly to bottom, sides, and rim of pan (volume will decrease after crust is evenly distributed and pressed into place). Place in freezer for 15 minutes.
3. Preheat oven to 400 degrees. Cover crust loosely with aluminum

foil. Place in center section of oven and bake for 10 minutes. Transfer to rack to cool. Crust will firm up when cooled.

4. To prepare filling, drain juice from canned pineapple into a heavy-bottomed saucepan. Place pineapples in large bowl. To saucepan, add concentrate, lemon juice, and nutmeg, stirring to blend. Sprinkle with gelatin and let stand for 3 minutes to soften.

5. Place saucepan over moderate heat. Whisk in 1 egg yolk, sugar, and honey. Bring to simmering point. Whisk and cook until mixture lightly coats a spoon (about 8 minutes). Stir in strawberries. Cook until berries are completely thawed (about 3 minutes). Remove from heat. Let cool completely.

6. To pineapples, add the cheese and milk, stirring to combine. When strawberry medley has cooled, stir into cheese mixture. Place in refrigerator and chill for 20 minutes. Stir. Return to refrigerator and chill until uniformly thickened but not set.

7. Whip egg whites until stiff. Stir ¼ into thickened mixture; fold in balance. Chill for 10 minutes.

8. Pile into prepared shell, mounding in center, and spreading to within ½ inch from edge of crust. Smooth out with spatula. Chill for at least 3 hours before serving.

Yield: **Serves 8**

Note: Choose graham crackers that are made without palm oils and/ or hydrogenated fats. Break up about 12 crackers and pulverize in food blender or processor.

STRAWBERRY CHEESE PIE

It tastes very much like rich, creamy Italian cheesecake, but the filling is based on unsalted dry-curd cottage cheese that contains only ½ percent fat! The rich taste comes from small amounts of cream, light cream cheese, and light sour cream. The filling, in a crisp pie shell, is topped with a sweet strawberry glaze. Light, of course.

For the crust and filling:

1 recipe crust from Tutti-Frutti
    Chiffon Pie (page 194)
2 12-ounce boxes unsalted dry-curd
    cottage cheese (½% milk
    fat)
3 tablespoons whipping cream
⅔ cup Light Choice sour cream
6 ounces light cream cheese
    (Neufchâtel)
2½ teaspoons finely minced lemon

zest
3 eggs, separated (see Note)
½ teaspoon each ground
    cardamom and cinnamon
6 tablespoons sugar
½ teaspoon pure vanilla extract
3 tablespoons unbleached flour,
    sifted
¼ teaspoon cream of tartar

For the glaze:

1 10-ounce box frozen strawberries
    in syrup
½ teaspoon freshly grated nutmeg
2 tablespoons fresh lemon juice

1 tablespoon cornstarch
2 tablespoons orange liqueur or
    cognac

1. Prepare crust first, following directions through Step 2. Let stand at room temperature while filling is prepared. Preheat oven to 300 degrees.
2. Spread cheese across large nonstick skillet. Place over medium-high heat and cook while stirring for 5 minutes. Liquid will exude from solids. Pour contents of skillet into strainer and drain, pressing out as much liquid as you can. Let cool for 5 minutes. Transfer to workbowl of food processor that has been fitted with steel blade. Add whipping cream and sour cream. Process until very smooth. Stop machine. Add cream cheese and lemon zest. Process for 4 seconds. Stop machine.
3. Drop in egg yolks, spices, 3 tablespoons sugar, and vanilla extract. Process for 15 seconds. Scrape into a large bowl. Using a wooden spoon, fold in flour.

4. Using large whisk of mixing machine, whip egg whites on moderate speed until foamy. With machine running, sprinkle in remaining 3 tablespoons sugar, and cream of tartar. Increase speed and beat until glossy peaks form (do not overbeat).

5. Stir about ¾ cup beaten whites into yolk batter; fold in balance. Pile into prepared shell, mounding in center and spreading to within ½ inch from edge of crust. Smooth out with spatula. Bake in center section of oven for 50 minutes. Pie will puff up. Partially open oven door, wedging if necessary to hold. Let pie cool in oven for 45 minutes. The center will recede slightly. Remove from oven and place on rack to cool completely.

6. To make glaze, place berries in a small enameled saucepan. Cover and cook over low heat until defrosted. Add nutmeg and lemon juice and cook, uncovered, for 2 minutes. Put cornstarch in a cup. While stirring with a small spoon, add liqueur slowly, blending until very smooth. Drizzle into berries. Cook over moderate heat until thickened (about 1½ minutes), stirring frequently. To hasten cooling, pour glaze into a small bowl and refrigerate. Spread onto pie. Chill pie for 2 hours before serving.

Yield: **Serves 8**

Note: Cholesterol watchers, don't let the egg yolks frighten you. They contribute only about 90 milligrams of cholesterol per serving.

FROZEN CHOCOLATE CAKE ROLL

Rich chocolate cake, filled with whipped cream or butter cream and spiraled in jelly-roll fashion, is an American favorite—and a dieter's nightmare. This version looks as rich and beautiful as the original, but it has none of the ingredients that make health-conscious people quiver.

1/4 cup cake flour (not self-rising)
1/4 teaspoon salt
1 1/2 teaspoons sweet
    butter/margarine blend
1 recipe Creamy Topping (page
    202)
2/3 cup unsweetened carob chips
    (available in health-food
    stores)
5 teaspoons unsweetened cocoa

1 tablespoon freeze-dried coffee,
    regular or decaffeinated
3 tablespoons frozen apple juice
    concentrate
1 teaspoon pure vanilla extract
6 eggs (use 3 yolks and 6 whites),
    room temperature
1/2 cup superfine sugar
3 tablespoons confectioner's sugar

1. Preheat oven to 350 degrees. Sift flour and salt into a small bowl. Grease a 10 × 15-inch jelly-roll pan with shortening. Line with wax paper, smoothing evenly across bottom and pressing against the sides of the pan. Grease the paper as far as 1 inch up the sides of the pan. Set aside.

2. Proceed with Steps 1 and 2 of the recipe for Creamy Topping, using the basic recipe or any variation.

3. In the top of a double boiler, combine carob chips, 3 teaspoons cocoa, coffee, and concentrate. Cook over simmering water, stirring continuously, until chips melt and mixture is smooth. Remove from heat and stir in vanilla extract.

4. Drop 3 egg yolks into a large mixing bowl. (Place whites in mixing machine bowl.) Whisk or beat yolks until light. Gradually whisk or beat in 1/4 cup sugar until lemon-colored and smooth. Whisk or beat in carob until glossy. Stir in the flour mix.

5. Beat egg whites on medium speed until foamy. Increase speed and continue beating until thick. With machine running at high speed, sprinkle in remaining 1/4 cup sugar, a little at a time. Continue beating whites until glossy and firm (about 4 minutes). With a wooden spoon, stir 1/4 cup beaten whites briskly into the cocoa mixture. Tilt bowl and fold in remaining whites carefully.

6. Turn into the prepared pan, spreading batter across pan evenly with flexible spatula. Bake in center section of oven until firm to the touch and toothpick inserted comes out clean (15 to 18 minutes). Remove pan from oven and place on rack. Cover tautly with clean dishcloth. Sprinkle cloth with water. Let cake cool for 30 minutes.
7. Ten minutes before cake finishes cooling, complete the recipe for Creamy Topping. Place in freezer until ready to use.
8. Combine remaining 2 teaspoons cocoa with confectioner's sugar. Sprinkle half the mixture over the cooled cake. Place a long sheet of wax paper over the cake and carefully invert onto firm surface. Peel off baked-on paper. Cut away crisp edges.
9. Spread half the topping to within ½ inch from edges. (Freeze remaining topping.) Roll up carefully, supporting the cake with paper while rolling. Transfer to a large serving plate. Mask cracks (there will be some) with dabs of topping. Then sprinkle all over with the balance of the cocoa mix. Turn freezer up to high. Freeze cake for 2 hours before slicing with sharp serrated knife. If cake remains in freezer more than 2 hours, place in refrigerator for 15 minutes before serving.

Yield: **Serves 8**

Note: Cholesterol watchers, don't let the egg yolks frighten you. There are only about 90 milligrams of cholesterol per serving.

SPICED APRICOT LOAF

I've made a purée from tangy dried apricots sweetened with a touch of honey. Most of it is beaten into a thrice-sifted flour and spice batter; the remainder is pushed into the middle of the loaf. See the variation, too, for a jamlike spread that's delicious over breakfast toast.

4 ounces unsulphured dried apricot halves (available in health-food stores)
About 1 1/4 cups water
2 tablespoons plus 2 teaspoons flavorful honey
2 cups unbleached flour
2 1/2 teaspoons non-aluminum baking powder
1/8 teaspoon salt
1/2 teaspoon each ground coriander, ginger, and cardamom

1/4 cup sweet butter/margarine blend
3 tablespoons sugar
3 tablespoons frozen apple juice concentrate
2 large eggs
1/2 teaspoon each pure vanilla extract and almond extract
6 tablespoons Light Choice sour cream
1/4 cup milk (1% milk fat)
2 tablespoons confectioner's sugar

1. Preheat oven to 350 degrees. Put apricots in colander. Rinse under cold running water. Transfer to small enameled saucepan. Add just enough water to cover; soak for 10 minutes. Place over high heat. Bring to a boil. Reduce heat to a slow boil and cook, uncovered, until most of liquid is evaporated and fruit is soft. (One cup of mixture should remain in saucepan.) Stir in honey; let cool for 5 minutes. Purée in food processor or blender. Transfer to a cup and set aside.
2. Sift flour, baking powder, salt, and spices 3 times. Set aside.
3. In large bowl of mixing machine, combine shortening, sugar, and concentrate. Beat on medium-high speed of mixing machine until the consistency of small-curd cottage cheese. Beat in eggs, one at a time. Then spoon in all but 1/4 cup puree and extracts. Beat until well blended.
4. While beating, spoon in 1 tablespoon sour cream at a time; then slowly add sifted dry ingredients alternately with milk. Beat on medium speed for 1 minute.
5. Grease an 8- or 9-inch loaf pan lightly with sweet butter/margarine blend. Fill with batter. Place teaspoons of remaining apricot purée lengthwise down center of cake. With knife, depress purée so that it

settles into batter. Dribble remaining 2 teaspoons honey down center of cake over purée. Give pan one sharp rap to disperse air bubbles. Place in center section of oven and bake for 45 minutes. Place pan on rack to cool for 5 minutes.

6. Sprinkle and spread confectioner's sugar across sheet of wax paper. Invert cake onto paper, then stand it upright on paper so that remaining sugar coats bottom of cake. Place on rack and let cool to room temperature before slicing.

Yield: **10 to 12 slices**

Variations:

1. Follow instructions in Step 1, adding ¼ teaspoon each ground cardamom and coriander *before* cooking apricots, and 3 tablespoons flavorful honey *after* mixture is puréed. Use as a jamlike spread.

2. Serve as a topping. Complete Variation 1 and stir in 2 tablespoons Light Choice sour cream or plain low-fat yogurt. Serve with Sweet Pancake Puffs or New-Style Griddle Cakes (pages 212 and 209).

CREAMY TOPPING (OR AIRY ICE-MILK)

This is a delectable zabaglione-like topping, which, when frozen, becomes a luscious ice-milk. Enjoy it often because it contains *no* fat and loads of health-essential calcium. It's also easy to make, and the variations are almost endless.

3/4 cup evaporated skim milk (see Note)
3 tablespoons each frozen orange and apple juice concentrate
1/2 teaspoon each ground ginger and cinnamon

1/4 teaspoon ground cardamom or coriander
2 tablespoons superfine sugar
1 tablespoon flavorful honey
1 teaspoon fresh lemon juice
1 teaspoon pure vanilla extract

1. Pour milk into large mixing machine bowl. Place bowl and whisk attachment in freezer. Chill until center is almost frozen (about 50 minutes).
2. In medium freeze-proof container, combine frozen concentrate, spices, sugar, and honey. Place in freezer.
3. Attach cold whisk attachment to mixing machine. Whip almost-frozen milk on high speed for 1 minute. Sprinkle in lemon juice and beat until stiff as whipped cream (4 to 5 minutes). With machine running, spoon in frozen juice mixture and vanilla extract. Beat on high speed until firm peaks form (3 to 4 minutes). Serve immediately as a dessert, spooned into chilled decorative dishes; or over fruit, pies, or cakes.
4. To serve as ice-milk, transfer to freeze-proof containers, leaving a 1-inch space at the top, and freeze for 2 to 3 hours for a frozen custard consistency and 4 to 5 hours for an airy-textured consistency. (The efficiency of your freezer will determine freezing time.) Leftovers may be stored in freezer. Place in refrigerator to soften 1 hour before serving.

Yield: **About 6 cups**

Note: Evaporated skim milk, manufactured by PET and labeled PET LIGHT, is recommended because it's the only evaporated skim milk that I know of that beats to the consistency of whipped cream. However, any other brand of evaporated skim milk may be used for recipes where no whipping is indicated.

Variations:

1. Substitute frozen pineapple juice concentrate for apple juice concentrate; substitute ½ teaspoon almond extract for vanilla extract.
2. For a coffee-flavored topping, in a small saucepan, heat and dissolve 3 tablespoons freeze-dried decaffeinated or regular coffee (or coffee substitute) in ¼ cup apple juice with 1 tablespoon flavorful honey. Let cool. Add to frozen concentrates in Step 2.
3. For a chocolate topping, in small heavy-bottomed saucepan, combine 2 tablespoons frozen concentrates with 1½ squares unsweetened chocolate, 1 teaspoon each cinnamon and cardamom (or coriander), 3 tablespoons superfine sugar, and honey. Cook and stir over low heat until chocolate dissolves completely. Cool. Pour into freeze-proof container with remaining 4 tablespoons combined concentrates and place in freezer (Step 2). Continue with Step 3, eliminating spices, sugar, and honey.
4. For a raspberry/chocolate ripple, prepare the recipe for my Raspberry/Chocolate Sauce (page 208). Pour sauce into freeze-proof container and chill until thickened but not frozen. When basic dessert is fully whipped and recipe completed, dribble in mixture. Using a wooden spoon, fold over once or twice without blending.
5. This creamy-smooth variation is a cousin to ice cream. It includes some fat, but far less than you'll find in any commercial ice cream. In place of ¾ cup evaporated skim milk, use ½ cup. Beat until stiff according to instructions in Steps 1 through 3. Include ¼ cup whipping cream in variation. To whip, chill bowl and whipping attachment. Pour cream into bowl and beat until stiff. Fold into beaten milk mixture.

CHOCOLATE/CHESTNUT MOUSSE

Most Americans are unaware of the low-calorie, low-fat content of chestnuts. Though they're filling when roasted and eaten whole, one nut has a mere 14 calories with a scant 0.1 percent fat, most of which is "good fat" (polyunsaturated). With these stunning health features in mind, I've combined chestnuts with a hint of chocolate to give you a sumptuous melt-in-your-mouth dessert. I prefer canned French marrons (they're naturally sweeter than their American cousin) and whole chestnuts (because they have more flavor than the purée).

¾ cup evaporated skim milk (see Note for Creamy Topping, page 202)
¼ cup water
2 packets plain gelatin
1 15½-ounce can imported whole peeled chestnuts, packed in water
1 square unsweetened chocolate
4 tablespoons frozen orange juice concentrate

½ teaspoon each freshly grated nutmeg and cinnamon
2 tablespoons flavorful honey, such as thyme
2 eggs (use 1 yolk and 2 whites)
1 teaspoon pure vanilla extract
1 to 2 tablespoons orange liqueur or cognac (optional)
1 teaspoon fresh lemon juice
¼ teaspoon cream of tartar
3 tablespoons superfine sugar

1. Pour ½ cup evaporated skim milk into large mixing machine bowl. Place bowl and whisk attachment in freezer. Chill until center is almost frozen (about 50 minutes).
2. Pour water into a cup. Sprinkle with gelatin. Stir. Let stand for 5 minutes.
3. Pick out 5 firm chestnut halves to use as garnish. Pour remaining contents of can and reserved ¼ cup milk into food blender. Blend on high speed until completely smooth. (You may have to stop the blender once or twice to stir up mixture from bottom.) Scrape into large bowl. Set aside.
4. Half-fill the bottom section of a double boiler with water. Bring to a boil. Put chocolate and 2 tablespoons concentrate into top section. Place over heat and melt. Reduce heat. Whisk in softened gelatin. Cook for 1 minute. Add spices and honey. Whisk and cook for 1 minute.
5. Drop egg yolk into a cup (and egg whites into another large mixing

machine bowl). Beat yolk with fork. While whisking, dribble into hot mixture. Cook for 3 minutes. Whisk into chestnut purée with remaining 2 tablespoons concentrate and vanilla extract. Stir in liqueur if desired. Set aside.

6. Attach cold whisk attachment to mixing machine. Beat almost-frozen milk on high speed for 1 minute. Sprinkle in lemon juice and beat until stiff as whipped cream. Whisk ¼ into purée; fold in remainder. Rinse and dry whisk attachment.

7. Beat egg whites on medium speed until foamy. Add cream of tartar. Turn up to highest speed. Sprinkle in sugar, a little at a time. Beat until firm and glossy, taking care not to overbeat. Fold into mousse, tilting bowl to ease folding motion. Pile into chilled decorative glass serving bowl, smoothing out top. Garnish with reserved chestnuts. Chill for 1 hour for a creamy soft texture, or 3 hours or longer for a firmer texture.

Yield: **10 or more servings**

SHERRIED APPLESAUCE

My version of this familiar kitchen staple is flavored with fruit juice, raisins, sweet spices, and the essence of sophisticated dry sherry. Try it with Tofu Potato Pancakes (page 51) for lunch.

6 crisp, sweet apples, scrubbed,
    cored, and sliced (about 2 1/2
    pounds)
1/2 cup raisins
3 tablespoons frozen pineapple juice
    concentrate
3/4 cup unsweetened apple juice

1/4 cup dry sherry
4 whole cloves
1/2 teaspoon each ground
    cardamom and cinnamon
1/4 teaspoon allspice
Up to 2 tablespoons sugar or honey
    (optional)

1. Combine first 6 ingredients in a 2 1/2- to 3-quart saucepan. Bring to a boil. Reduce heat to simmering. Cover partially and cook until apples are tender when pierced with tip of a sharp knife (about 15 minutes, depending upon texture of fruit). Uncover and let cool for 5 minutes.
2. Transfer to food mill and purée into bowl. Stir in spices. Taste for sweetness, adding sugar or honey if desired. Store in a tightly closed glass jar for up to 1 week.

Yield: **3 cups; recipe may be doubled**

LIGHT RASPBERRY/BANANA ICE CREAM

The smoothness of this light ice cream is achieved by adding small amounts of whole milk and light cream to its base of evaporated skim milk. A true ice cream—but a light one!

1 12-ounce can evaporated skim
    milk
1 10-ounce box frozen raspberries
    in syrup, partially defrosted
1/2 cup mashed ripe banana
1/2 cup whole milk
3/4 cup light cream
1 tablespoon superfine sugar

1/4 teaspoon each freshly grated
    nutmeg, ground cardamom,
    and ground coriander
1 small egg yolk
2 teaspoons cornstarch, dissolved in
    2 teaspoons water
1/2 teaspoon almond extract

1. Pour evaporated skim milk into a large bowl. Stir in berries and banana. Place in refrigerator.
2. Half-fill the bottom of a double boiler with water. Bring to a boil. Reduce heat to simmering. In top section, combine whole milk, cream, sugar, and spices. Whisk and cook until just below boiling point.
3. In a cup, beat egg yolk lightly. While whisking, dribble it into pot. Cook for 5 minutes, whisking often. Dribble in cornstarch mixture. Whisk over simmering water until mixture coats a metal spoon (4 to 5 minutes). Remove from heat and let cool for 5 minutes.
4. Pour into chilled fruit medley. Stir in almond extract. Chill in freezer for 30 minutes. Then pour into ice-cream maker, following manufacturer's directions.

Yield: **About 1 quart**

STRAWBERRY ICE-MILK

The bright taste of fresh strawberries shines through this 0% fat ice-milk. Its main sweetening agents are apple juice and sweet spices, with only 3 tablespoons of sugar added instead of the usual 16 or more.

2 cups sliced fresh strawberries
1 cup unsweetened apple juice
1/2 teaspoon each freshly ground
   nutmeg and ground coriander
5 tablespoons fruit juice–sweetened
   strawberry conserves
3 tablespoons superfine sugar
3 cups evaporated skim milk,
   chilled
1/4 teaspoon almond extract

1. Combine strawberries, apple juice, and spices in a small heavy-bottomed saucepan. Bring to a boil. Reduce heat to simmering and cook, uncovered, for 1 1/2 minutes. Stir in conserves and sugar. Chill.
2. Pour milk into a large bowl. Stir in strawberry mix and almond extract. Turn into ice-cream maker, following manufacturer's instructions.

Yield: **1 quart**

Note: Because there is no fat in this ice-milk, it will become hard when frozen for longer than 12 hours. To soften, transfer from freezer to refrigerator 1 hour before serving.

RASPBERRY/CHOCOLATE SAUCE

Raspberries and chocolate love each other. This version *tastes* sinfully delicious, but only a small amount of sweetener is used, and the creaminess is derived from thick evaporated skim milk. Slightly tart, it complements myriad cakes and ice creams (see *Serving suggestion*).

1 12-ounce bag unsweetened frozen raspberries
2 tablespoons each sugar and flavorful honey
1 square unsweetened chocolate
3 tablespoons frozen pineapple juice concentrate
3 tablespoons evaporated skim milk
¼ teaspoon ground cardamom
½ teaspoon pure vanilla extract

1. Place frozen berries in heavy-bottomed 2-quart saucepan. Cook, covered, over low heat until berries give up their liquid (about 10 minutes), stirring from time to time. Place fine-meshed strainer (not a sieve) over a bowl. Using a large spoon stir in circular motion, pressing against strainer, to exude all juice and pulp from raspberries. Stir in sugar and honey while warm. Set aside. Rinse out saucepan.
2. Add chocolate and concentrate to saucepan. Cook, uncovered, over low heat until chocolate dissolves. Stir in milk and cardamom; cook for 1 minute. Using a rubber spatula, scrape mixture into raspberry purée. Stir in vanilla extract. Pour into a large jar and chill.

Yield: **1½ cups**

Serving suggestion: To create an Outrageous Cake à la Mode, arrange 4 slices of Angelic Sponge Cake or Spiced Apricot Loaf (pages 190, 200) on a large flat plate. Spoon each slice with ¼ cup sauce, letting it absorb into cake. Drizzle 1 teaspoon Grand Marnier liqueur over sauce. Top with Light Raspberry/Banana Ice Cream or Creamy Topping (pages 206, 202). Drizzle with a little more sauce. Sprinkle with chopped walnuts and serve at once.

NEW-STYLE GRIDDLE CAKES

To get the health benefits and pleasure of oat bran into your fiber diet, I've invented a totally new kind of griddle cake. Oat bran *and* tasty buckwheat are combined with sweet pineapple juice and sweet spices, and the mixture is held together with tangy buttermilk.

¼ cup oat bran
¼ cup buckwheat flour (available in health-food stores)
1 cup unbleached flour
1 ½ teaspoons non-aluminum baking powder
¼ teaspoon each ground cinnamon and coriander
⅛ teaspoon salt (optional)

2 tablespoons frozen pineapple juice concentrate
1 egg
1 tablespoon peanut oil, plus oil for sautéing
1 cup low-fat buttermilk, preferably without salt
½ cup evaporated skim milk

1. Prepare batter just before cooking. Put oat bran in food blender and pulverize. Transfer to a bowl. Sift in flours, baking powder, spices, and salt if desired.
2. In a small bowl, combine concentrate with egg and oil. Beat with a fork to blend. Stir in milks. Add to dry ingredients and stir until moist.
3. Prepare griddle cakes in 3 batches in a large nonstick skillet or a well-seasoned iron skillet, brushing ½ teaspoon oil across skillet before sautéing. Heat skillet until a drop of cold water dropped into it bounces off. Using a ¼-cup measure, pour enough batter into skillet to make 4 4-inch pancakes. Cook until bubbles form on top of pancakes. Turn and cook until lightly brown. Transfer to a warm plate. Prepare remaining griddle cakes in the same manner. Serve at once.

Yield: **12 griddle cakes**

Variation: To make Blueberry Pancakes, stir in ¾ cup rinsed and drained fresh blueberries at the end of Step 3 and add 1 teaspoon fresh lemon juice to recipe.

PEAR PAN PIE

This is an oven pancake that looks like a pie. Juicy Bosc pears are slightly caramelized in an iron skillet then in a spiced buttermilk batter. The crust becomes brown and crunchy in a hot oven while the center remains moist (as in all well-prepared pies). It's a stunner at the breakfast table—just the thing for a relaxed weekend breakfast.

2 tablespoons fresh lemon juice
3 firm Bosc pears, peeled,
    quartered, and thinly sliced
    (see Note)
2½ tablespoons sweet
    butter/margarine blend
3 tablespoons sugar
½ teaspoon each ground
    cardamom, cinnamon, and
    freshly grated nutmeg
2 eggs, separated
1 tablespoon flavorful honey

1 cup low-fat buttermilk, preferably
    without salt
¼ cup each unbleached flour and
    stone-ground whole wheat
    flour
½ teaspoon non-aluminum baking
    powder
Pinch cream of tartar
½ lemon
2 to 3 teaspoons confectioner's
    sugar
Lemon wedges

1. Pour lemon juice into a medium bowl. Add pears as they're sliced, turning to coat. In a well-seasoned 10-inch iron skillet, melt 1 tablespoon shortening over moderate heat. Raise heat slightly and cook until lightly browned. Stir in pears (including juice), 2 tablespoons sugar, and half the spice mix. Cook while stirring until fruit becomes lightly browned and juices become syrupy (about 8 minutes). Transfer to a small bowl. Preheat oven to 400 degrees.
2. In a large bowl, whisk egg yolks, remaining 1 tablespoon sugar, remaining spices, and honey. Then gradually whisk in buttermilk until very smooth. Sift flours and baking powder into mix. Stir until well blended.
3. Beat egg whites on medium speed until foamy. Sprinkle in cream of tartar and beat on highest speed until stiff but not dry. Stir one-third into batter; fold in remainder. Batter will be light and fluffy.
4. Heat remaining 1½ tablespoons shortening in skillet over medium-high heat until lightly browned. Pour in batter, spreading to edges of pan and smoothing out top. Reduce heat to medium and cook for 1 minute. Spoon pears and their juices over batter, leaving a 1-inch border. Cook for 1 minute. Place skillet in center section of oven and bake for 15 minutes. Sprinkle with juice from ½ lemon; return to oven for 5 minutes.

5. Place pie on trivet at serving table and sprinkle with confectioner's sugar. Let cool for 5 minutes before slicing (center will recede slightly). Serve with lemon wedges.

Yield: **Serves 6**

Note: Bosc pears are usually picked and transported before they have ripened, arriving at your market rock-hard. Soften them to near-ripeness by placing in a paper bag with the top folded over for two days. They'll still be firm enough to retain their shape throughout the baking process.

BANANA FRENCH TOAST

Sweet, cake-textured Anadama Oatmeal Bread, saturated with a mix of ripe banana, evaporated skim milk, sweet spices, two egg whites, and just one egg yolk makes a light-as-a-cloud French toast.

4 1/2-inch slices Anadama Oatmeal
    Bread (page 160)
2 eggs (use 1 yolk and 2 whites)
1/4 teaspoon each ground
    coriander, cinnamon, and
    ground cardamom
1/4 cup milk

About 1/2 cup evaporated skim
    milk
1/2 ripe banana, sliced
Pinch salt
1 1/2 teaspoons each sweet
    butter/margarine blend and
    peanut oil

1. Cut each slice of bread in half. Place in a wide bowl.
2. Drop eggs into food blender. Add spices, milks, banana, and salt. Purée until very smooth. Pour half the mixture over bread. Shift slices and soak with remaining liquid, adding more milk if necessary to saturate bread completely. Let stand for 5 minutes.
3. Heat shortening and oil in a large nonstick skillet until hot. Add bread, pouring any unabsorbed liquid over slices. Cook over medium-high heat on each side until browned. Serve immediately; it won't wait!

Yield: **Serves 4**

SWEET PANCAKE PUFFS

These are raised breakfast pancakes, thicker and more cakelike than those in a typical stack. Your success with them depends largely on two factors: the even heat of the skillet and a watchful eye.

¼ buckwheat flour (available in health-food stores)
¾ cup unbleached flour
¼ teaspoon each ground ginger, coriander, and cinnamon
1 teaspoon non-aluminum baking powder
½ cup mashed ripe banana (1 medium banana)
2 eggs, separated (use 1 yolk and 2 whites)
2 tablespoons frozen pineapple juice

concentrate
1 tablespoon flavorful honey, such as thyme
1 cup whole milk or low-fat milk (1% milk fat)
2 teaspoons melted sweet butter/margarine blend
Pinch cream of tartar
About 1 tablespoon peanut oil
About 1 tablespoon confectioner's sugar
Fresh lemon juice

1. Sift first 4 listed ingredients into large bowl. In smaller bowl, combine and blend banana, 1 egg yolk, concentrate, and honey. Then whisk in milk and melted shortening. Stir into flour mix.
2. In large bowl of a mixing machine, using wire whisk attachment, beat egg whites on moderate speed until foamy. Add cream of tartar. Increase to highest speed and beat until firm and glossy (do not overbeat). Stir one-quarter into batter; fold in remainder.
3. Using a large nonstick skillet, prepare pancakes in batches. Brush skillet with film of oil. Place over moderate heat. When hot, brush again with oil. Scoop up scant quarter-cup of batter for each puff and drop into pan. Spread out gently to 4-inch diameter with spatula. Cook for 2 minutes. Brush film of oil between pancakes and tilt pan from side to side. Turn and cook for 2 minutes, or until golden brown, adjusting heat when necessary to prevent burning.
4. Serve puffs as they're made, with a dusting of confectioner's sugar and sprinklings of lemon juice.

Yield: **About 16 4-inch pancake puffs**

Variation: Substitute frozen orange juice concentrate for pineapple juice concentrate and use ½ teaspoon each ground cardamom and cinnamon in place of listed spices.

13

MY SEVEN-DAY MENU PLAN AND HOLIDAY MEAL

The menu plans that follow are suggestions. Mix them up, use them to inspire your own creative ideas, or tailor a menu plan to your family's tastes. One easy way to elaborate on this plan is to substitute similar foods—one of my soups for another of my soups, for example.

The Surgeon General's Report urges most Americans to cut down on calories, and my menu plan does just that. Eating the Diet for Life way may permit you to reach your ideal weight without feeling you're on a diet.

Most of my recipes serve four, so they're right for most family breakfasts and dinners. But today when lunch is eaten at home, it's usually for one, and that's what the Menu Plan calls for. On weekends and holidays, the lunch menu can be multiplied to serve the entire family (for mini-recipes just multiply ingredients by the number of servings). Most dinner leftovers retain their taste during an overnight stay in the fridge, and can be reheated for lunch. This is particularly true of soup leftovers—which are light and satisfying for midday eating, but meat and poultry fare well too. Next-day fish, though, fares better as a salad or a cold sandwich filling than as a reheated dish.

As for beverages, some coffee is okayed by Dr. Koop, and there's no warning against tea, so they can accompany your meals. Low-fat and skim milk are fine too. But Dr. Koop advises you to cut down your alcohol intake to about two drinks daily. One drink is defined as a 12-ounce beer, a 5-ounce glass of wine, or 1½ fluid ounces (1 jigger) of distilled spirits, each of which contains about ½ ounce of alcohol. (There's no limit on cooking with wine, because the heat evaporates the alcohol, leaving just the flavor.)

The menus are marked Day One, Day Two, and so on for identification purposes. There's no reason for you to follow them consecutively. Select your own sequence. I like to set up an alternating pattern for my main protein dish of the day: meat one day, fish the next, poultry the next, then repeat. Protein-food servings, in compliance with the National Research Council's recommendation, are usually about 3 to 3½ ounces. (Remember: There's about a 25 percent weight shrinkage from uncooked to cooked meat, fish, and poultry.)

Most important: Don't think you have to go through the whole seven days meal by meal. Just a meal or two a week is a good start, or even just a few dishes. I hope you'll find the Diet for Life way of cooking and eating habit-forming.

NOTE: Italicized titles are recipes featured in this book.

DAY ONE

Breakfast:

Melon wedges
New-Style Griddle Cakes (3 per serving)
Fruit juice–sweetened jelly or honey (1½ teaspoons per
    serving) *or*
Apricot Topping (see *Note 2* for *Apricot Loaf,* page 201)

Lunch:

Any of my *Soups* (1 cup per serving)
Club Sandwiches, 1 each, consisting of:
  · 3 thin slices of any of my *Breads,* bottom slice spread with:
  · 1 teaspoon *Low-Cholesterol Mayonnaise,* covered with
  · 3 ounces cooked sliced chicken, fish, or lean meat
  top section filled with:
  · *Savoy Salad* (drained)
Fresh fruit (1 piece per serving)

Dinner:

Watercress and Mushroom Salad with *Oat Crackers*
Shrimp and Scallops in Saffron Sauce
Steamed rice
Carrot/Cauliflower Purée
Tutti-Frutti Chiffon Pie (1 wedge per serving)

DAY TWO

Breakfast:

Fresh fruit juice of your choice (1 cup per serving)
Pear Pan Pie (1 wedge per serving)

Lunch:

Salad Plate (per serving), consisting of:
 · Crisp green lettuce
 · *Oat Crackers* (4 or 5), or
 · *Breakfast or Dinner Cornbread* (2 squares per serving)
topped generously with *Fruit and Nut Cheese Spread*
surrounded with
 · Radish rosettes
 · Cucumber slices
moistened with
 · *Buttermilk Salad Dressing* (up to 2 tablespoons per serving)
Angelic Sponge Cake (1 serving)

Dinner:

Mixed Salad with Carrot Juice Vinaigrette
Lemon Chicken with Porcini Mushrooms
Wild Rice and Barley Medley
Steamed peas, seasoned with:
 · minced fresh mint
 · freshly grated nutmeg
 · pinch of salt (if desired)
 · sweet butter/margarine blend (1 teaspoon per serving)
Chocolate/Chestnut Mousse (¾ cup per serving)

DAY THREE

Breakfast:

Fresh orange sections (1 orange per serving)
Pancake Puffs (4 per serving)
Fruit juice–sweetened jelly (up to 2 teaspoons per serving)

Lunch:

Quick Pasta with Julienne Chicken (to serve 1), consisting of:
 · 3 ounces boned and skinned chicken breasts cut into
¼-inch strips
sprinkled and rubbed with mixture of:
 · ¼ teaspoon mild curry powder
 · ¼ teaspoon dried tarragon leaves
 · dash of salt
sautéed over medium-high heat in small nonstick skillet for 5
minutes with:
 · 1 teaspoon Italian olive oil;
then add

- ½ cup my *Tomato Sauce;*
  simmer until heated through, then pour over
- 1 ounce just-cooked vermicelli or capellini sprinkled with
- 2 teaspoons freshly grated Parmesan cheese and
- minced parsley

Fresh fruit (1 serving)

Dinner:

Warm Radicchio Salad
Sautéed Steak with Onion Marmalade
Oven-Baked Potato Pancakes
Fresh berries (½ cup per serving), spooned with:
- *Creamy Topping* (up to ½ cup per serving)

DAY FOUR

Breakfast:

Baked apple (1 apple per serving), cored, filled with mixture of:
- ¼ cup raisins
- ¼ teaspoon each cinnamon and ground cardamom or coriander
- 1 teaspoon brown sugar
- 2 tablespoons unsweetened apple juice

Cooked oatmeal (1 cup per serving), served with:
- ¼ cup undiluted evaporated skim milk (deliciously sweet without added sugar)

Morning Cake Bread (1 slice per serving)

Lunch:

Pumpkin Soup (1 cup per serving)
Tofu Potato Pancakes (4 per serving), garnished with crisp arugula or watercress
Spiced Applesauce (up to ¾ cup per serving)

Dinner:

Eggplant Munchies
Sophisticated Catfish
Light Corn Pudding
Steamed minted green beans (to serve 4),
  consisting of:
- ¾ pound fresh green beans, julienned, steamed, moistened with
- 2 teaspoons sweet butter/margarine blend, sprinkled with

- ¼ teaspoon freshly grated nutmeg
- 1 tablespoon minced fresh mint
- pinch salt

Apricot Loaf (1 slice per serving)

DAY FIVE

Breakfast:

Fresh berries (½ cup per serving), sweetened to taste with mixture of:
- ¼ teaspoon cinnamon
- 2 tablespoons unsweetened apple juice, topped with
- plain low-fat yogurt (½ cup per serving), sweetened with
- flavorful honey, if desired (1 teaspoon per serving)

Curried scrambled eggs, prepared in nonstick skillet with:
- 1 teaspoon sweet butter/margarine blend
- 4 eggs (use 2 yolks, 4 whites), beaten with
- ⅛ teaspoon salt
- ¼ teaspoon mild curry powder
- 2 tablespoons undiluted evaporated skim milk

2 thin slices any of my *Breads,* or 1 of my *Muffins* per serving

Lunch:

Clear consommé (1 cup per serving)

Fresh fish fillet (4 ounces, uncooked, per serving), seasoned with:
- fresh lemon juice
- 1 teaspoon sweet butter/margarine blend,

then broiled under high heat for 3 minutes and spread with
- about 2½ tablespoons of *Barbecue Sauce,* and broiled for 2 minutes

2 slices *Sourdough French Bread*

Oatmeal Chip Cookies (2 per serving)

Dinner:

Madeira Duxelles on *Oat Crackers*
Oven-"Fried" Chicken
Sautéed Zucchini with Horseradish
Mixed Green Salad with *Buttermilk Salad Dressing* (2 tablespoons per serving)
Light Raspberry/Banana Ice Cream (½ cup per serving)

DAY SIX

Breakfast:

Apricot Purée (¼ cup per serving)—see Step 1 of recipe for
Apricot Loaf (page 200)—spooned with:
  · milk (skim, 1% fat, or undiluted evaporated skim milk), to
    taste
Choice of any of my *Muffins,* spread with:
  · low-fat cottage cheese, and
  · fruit juice–sweetened jelly, if desired (up to 2 teaspoons per
    serving)

Lunch:

Veal scaloppine with jalapeño pepper, consisting of:
  · 4 ounces tender veal scaloppine (per serving), sprinkled
    and rubbed with
  · 1 teaspoon *Savory Seasoning,*
  then quickly sautéed in nonstick skillet with
  · 1 teaspoon Italian olive oil
  · 1 teaspoon *Vegetable Mix*
  · ½ to 1 teaspoon minced jalapeño pepper
Savoy Salad (¾ cup per serving)
1 or 2 slices any of my *Breads*
Fresh fruit (1 piece per serving)

Dinner:

Pinto Bean Cakes, served on a bed of Romaine lettuce and
  chopped scallion
Golden Carrot Soup with Shrimp (1¼ cups per serving)
Sweet Buns (1 per serving)
Frozen Chocolate Cake Roll (1 slice per serving)

DAY SEVEN

Breakfast:

Broiled grapefruit (½ grapefruit per serving), spooned before
  broiling with mixture of:
  · ¼ teaspoon each cinnamon and ground cardamom or
    coriander
  · 2 teaspoons brown sugar or flavorful honey
  · ¼ cup unsweetened pineapple juice
Banana French Toast (1 whole slice per serving)
Fruit juice–sweetened jelly (up to 2 teaspoons per serving)

Lunch:

Carrot/tomato juice cocktail (1 cup per serving), consisting of:
  · ½ cup each unseasoned carrot juice and tomato juice
  · Worcestershire sauce to taste
Lentil/Bulgur Salad (up to ¾ cup per serving), spooned on a
  bed of:
    · crisp salad greens, garnished with
    · radish rosettes and sliced cucumbers
Oatmeal Chip Cookies with Apricots (2 per serving)

Dinner:

Sun-Dried Tomato Tart
Bok Choy Salad
Curried Halibut Fillets
Strawberry Ice-Milk (¾ cup per serving)

HOLIDAY MEAL

Green Pea and Watercress Soup
Shrimp-filled Crepes
Holiday Cornish Hens with *Hot Cranberry Sauce*
Potato and Apple Medley
Steamed Baby Vegetables, consisting of:
    · 1 pound assorted baby vegetables
    · 1 cup white turnip, cut in ½-inch cubes
    seasoned with
    · 1 tablespoon sweet butter/margarine blend
    · ¼ teaspoon freshly grated nutmeg
    · ¼ teaspoon salt
    · freshly ground black or white pepper
    · 2 tablespoons just-snipped dill or coarsely chopped fresh corian-
      der
Delicate Apple/Cranberry Pie (1 wedge per serving)

AFTERTHOUGHTS

For numbers watchers, here is eating advice for a healthier diet issued in March 1989 by the Committee on Diet and Health of the National Research Council. Unlike the Surgeon General's recommendations, these include some specific amounts. My Menu Plan meets those numerical requirements, and in some cases beats them. Daily salt intake, for example, is far less than the recommended 4,500–6,000 milligram ceiling.

Alcohol: Reduce to at most 1 ounce of pure alcohol a day, equivalent to two cans of beer, two small glasses of wine, or two average cocktails. Consumption of any alcohol is not recommended.

Cholesterol: Reduce intake to less than 300 milligrams a day.

Complex carbohydrates: Consume about 55 percent of total calories.

Fat: Reduce intake of total fat to 30 percent of total calories, and of saturated fat to 10 percent.

Fiber: No specific recommendations.

Protein: Consume about 15 percent of total calories.

Salt: Reduce to less than 6,000 milligrams a day, but 4,500 milligrams or less is preferred.

Sugar: No specific recommendations.

Together, the Surgeon General's Report on Nutrition and Health (1988) and the Report of the National Research Council (1989) advise that a healthful diet may reduce the risks of cardiovascular diseases, cancer, diabetes, obesity, osteoporosis, dental caries (cavities), and chronic liver and kidney diseases. In 1988, a study conducted at the University of California, Berkeley, indicated that lifestyle changes alone, without drugs or surgery, could halt or reverse atherosclerosis that can lead to heart attack. The major components of such an altered lifestyle are *proper diet* and *exercise.*

For a copy of the Surgeon General's Report, write to the Superintendent of Documents, US Government Printing Office, Washington, DC 20402.

For a copy of the National Research Council's Report on Diet and Health, write to the National Academy Press, 2101 Constitution Avenue NW, Washington, DC 20418.

Both reports are available in complete and simplified versions. Write before ordering to obtain current prices.

Index